# BREAK FREE
## FROM
# OCD

**Dr Fiona Challacombe**
**Dr Victoria Bream Oldfield**
and **Professor Paul Salkovskis**

**Vermilion**
LONDON

7 9 10 8 6

Published in 2011 by Vermilion, an imprint of Ebury Publishing
Ebury Publishing is a Random House Group company

The Random House Group Limited Reg. No. 954009
Addresses for companies within the Random House Group can be found at
www.randomhouse.co.uk

A CIP catalogue record for this book is available from the British Library

The Random House Group Limited supports The Forest Stewardship
Council® (FSC®), the leading international forest-certification organisation.
Our books carrying the FSC label are printed on FSC®-certified paper.
FSC is the only forest-certification scheme supported by the leading
environmental organisations, including Greenpeace. Our
paper procurement policy can be found at
www.randomhouse.co.uk/environment

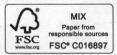

Printed and bound in Great Britain by Clays Ltd, St Ives PLC

ISBN 9780091939694

To buy books by your favourite authors and register for offers, visit www.rbooks.co.uk

The information in this book has been compiled by way of general guidance in
relation to the specific subjects addressed, but is not a substitute and not to be relied
on for medical, healthcare, pharmaceutical or other professional advice on specific
circumstances and in specific locations. Please consult your GP before changing,
stopping or starting any medical treatment. So far as the authors are aware the
information given is correct and up to date as at May 2011. Practice, laws and
regulations all change, and the reader should obtain up-to-date professional advice
on any such issues. The authors and publishers disclaim, as far as the law allows,
any liability arising directly or indirectly from the use, or misuse,
of the information contained in this book.

The case studies in this book are not from one person, but a compendium
of elements from the authors' experience of people with OCD.

**Dr Fiona Challacombe** MA (Cantab), DClinPsy, CPsychol, MBPS is a research fellow and clinical psychologist working at King's College London and the Centre for Anxiety Disorders and Trauma at the Maudsley Hospital, London. She is part of a national specialist service treating individuals with severe and complex OCD. Her research focuses on the impact of OCD on parenting and families, and investigating the delivery and refinement of cognitive behaviour therapy for OCD.

**Dr Victoria Bream Oldfield** MA (Oxon), DClinPsy, CPsychol, MBPS is a clinical psychologist working at the Centre for Anxiety Disorders and Trauma, Maudsley Hospital, London. She is part of a national specialist service treating individuals with severe and complex OCD. She studied experimental psychology at the University of Oxford, clinical psychology at the Institute of Psychiatry, King's College London, and trained in Cognitive Behaviour Therapy at the Oxford Cognitive Therapy Centre at the University of Oxford. Her research interests are in the phenomenology and treatment of OCD.

**Professor Paul Salkovskis** BSc, MPhil (Clin Psy), PhD, CPsychol, FBPS is Professor of Clinical Psychology and Applied Science and Programme Director of the forthcoming Doctorate programme in Clinical Psychology at the University of Bath. He is editor of the scientific journal *Behavioural and Cognitive Psychotherapy*. He has published over 250 scientific papers and recently received the Aaron T Beck award for contributions to cognitive therapy.

*To Isabella, Seraphina, Cora and Duncan*

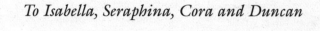

# CONTENTS

# ACKNOWLEDGEMENTS

We would like to thank all the people with OCD we have worked with over the years. The courage shown by those undertaking treatment and overcoming their difficulties continues to inspire us.

We would also like to thank our colleagues at the Centre for Anxiety Disorders and Trauma at the Maudsley Hospital, the University of Oxford and the Institute of Psychiatry, King's College London.

# HOW TO USE THIS BOOK

This book is a guide to self-help for people who already know or think they have obsessive–compulsive disorder (OCD). There are special sections aimed at friends and families who may want to read further into the book to gain knowledge of the problem and how to help (see pages 27–31 and 257–60).

OCD can come in many forms – if you have OCD we recommend reading about all the types of OCD described in this book. By gaining a really good understanding of how OCD works, you will get the best understanding of your own problems and how to beat them. We will move through thinking about the impact and the mechanics of the problem, and will use this information to help you both *know how to* and *choose to* change.

# 1

# WHAT IS OBSESSIVE–COMPULSIVE DISORDER?

In this chapter we will cover:

- The main features of obsessive–compulsive disorder
- Why it is normal to have 'intrusive thoughts' and how it is unhelpful to try to control them
- Why obsessive–compulsive disorder becomes a problem for some people
- Introduction to the 'cognitive behavioural' understanding of obsessive–compulsive disorder

Have you ever gone back to check that the gas is off, or thought that something is invisibly dirty or contaminated and taken extra care to clean it, or even thrown it away? Do you feel uncomfortable if your things aren't arranged in a very particular way? Have you ever had a thought that you might do something terrible and out of character? Have you had a thought or mental picture about something you think you should never think about? Ever noticed what seemed like an impulse to do something you don't really want to? Or had a 'bad' thought that you needed to cancel out in some way? These are all *intrusive thoughts*, meaning thoughts which pop into your head and *interrupt* what you are already thinking … they intrude! If they intrude so often and so strongly that they severely interfere with what you want to do, then you can be said to be suffering from obsessions and compulsions as a disorder: obsessive–compulsive disorder.

OCD has been increasingly mentioned in the media over the last few years, but not always correctly. Many people will have heard about the most common forms of the problem, affecting those who compulsively wash their hands or check things repeatedly, although there are many other types. However, precisely what drives people to get stuck in these patterns of thinking and behaving is not usually talked about, leading to misunderstanding of what the problem is. As a result, OCD can be offered as an explanation for almost anything which is repeated, from preferences for routine and order to the experience of everyday worries, or the motivation behind almost any 'quirky' behaviour which a person does more than once. Using everyday terminology, people with a strong interest are described as being 'obsessed' with it; people who are very focused are sometimes referred to as being 'obsessive'. Being strongly interested in something, or being perfectionistic and persistent about something important to you can be helpful in the right circumstances and may be enjoyable if these things happen by willing choice. However, *truly* obsessional behaviour is very different in that it is driven by personally unpleasant ideas linked to an uncomfortable or even unbearable feeling of anxiety, and stands apart from other kinds of 'obsessions' and compulsions in being neither helpful nor enjoyable. The person suffering from OCD does not feel that they have any choice about what is happening to them. However, we will show that the processes which drive OCD are all understandable as exaggerated versions of *normal* psychological experiences and worries which take hold and develop into OCD in certain people.

Sometimes, when seen from the outside, the problem of OCD can seem extreme, bizarre and so far from 'normality' as to appear 'mad'; this is, of course, one of the factors which stops people seeing the disorder for what it is and getting the right knowledge to fight the problem effectively. Unfortunately, this can also have the effect of cutting them off from seeking help (because they feel ashamed, scared or frightened of what will happen if they tell others). If you have OCD you may think of the problem as one of 'mad, bad or dangerous to know', all ideas that can fill you with some combination of shame, terror and misery. OCD is none of these things, and understanding how OCD works is an intrinsic part of moving through treatment and beating the problem so you can reclaim your life. Another factor which can interfere with how a person deals with OCD is when the problem becomes so completely consuming that the person loses their perspective. In this case, all you can think about is how to make sure that the things you fear do not happen. You become so taken up with what you are trying to do by washing, checking and other rituals that you are unable to see that your problem is fear of the thing which you are focused on, rather than the thing itself.

So, when people have OCD, the three most obvious elements of the way they experience it are:

1. Obsessional thoughts, impulses, images and doubts
2. Compulsions, both in terms of what people try to do and what they try to think
3. The impairment, distress and difficulty that they cause

## OBSESSIONS

Obsessions, also known as 'intrusive thoughts', are *unwanted and unacceptable* thoughts that seem to appear in your mind in an *unbidden* way. Obsessions can be *thoughts* in words but can also be *images, urges,* as if one wants to do something, or *feelings of doubt*. We will refer to them as 'thoughts' for clarity of writing from this point. Everyone has had the experience of a song coming into their head that stays around all day; when walking down the street many people experience nonsense phrases or perhaps swear words popping into their head. Unlike other thoughts that pass through our minds, obsessive thoughts are experienced as any or all of repugnant, senseless, unacceptable; they are always difficult to dismiss or ignore. Obsessional thoughts, therefore, seem to stand out from other sorts of thoughts because they are alien to the way we see ourselves. That is, they don't fit with who we think we are (but often people with OCD fear that they might reveal some terrible truth about themselves).

It would be impossible to list all the possible intrusive thoughts people could have as they are so many and varied. Here are some common intrusive thoughts, images and urges that we will revisit throughout the book:

## THOUGHTS
- 'There might be blood in my food'
- 'That is contaminated with germs'
- 'My appointment is on Friday 13th'
- 'Perhaps I am a rapist'

## DOUBTS
- 'Have I left the front door open?'
- 'Did I run someone over without realising it?'

## IMAGES
- Mum dead in a car crash
- Abusing a baby or child

## URGES
- 'I must touch that or I won't feel right'
- To jump in front of a train
- To physically assault someone

Looking at the list above, if you are someone who knows or thinks that they have OCD, you may have spotted a thought similar to one that particularly bothers you. There are probably others in the list that don't bother you, but would certainly be troublesome to someone else. Surprising as it may seem, there are people who may have had any one of the thoughts listed above, but are not particularly worried by them and certainly do not have OCD. In fact, **everyone has thoughts such as these**. Often people are surprised to find out that everyone has all sorts of intrusive thoughts – including the nasty ones: thoughts of harm coming to people, images of violence, urges to check things, doubts about whether they have done something or impulses to do something

---

**RESEARCH NOTE**

In the 1970s, when the cognitive understanding of OCD was being developed, two experts in OCD thought it was important to know whether 'normal' people had intrusive thoughts, and whether they were different in content from those that troubled people with OCD. They asked people with and without OCD to write down their intrusive thoughts and they mixed up the list. They then asked professionals with experience in working with OCD to say which had come from people with OCD and which had not. They were not able to tell the difference between normal intrusive thoughts and obsessional intrusive thoughts. Normal intrusive thoughts included:

- Impulse to hurt or harm someone
- I'll jump on the rails when the train approaches
- I feel really angry about what he did last year
- Image of daughter dying in a terrorist attack
- Thoughts of acts of violence during sex
- What if I have cancer?
- Urge to smash up possessions
- I am contaminated with asbestos
- Impulse to violently attack and kill a dog

Rachman, S. & De Silva, P. (1978), 'Normal and Abnormal Obsessions', *Behaviour Research and Therapy*, 16, 233–248.

---

they consider 'terrible'. For most people the thoughts just flicker in and out of their mind without causing the levels of distress seen in OCD.

The notion that 'intrusive thoughts' are everyday occurrences was backed up by research conducted in the late 1970s and 1980s which investigated whether there were differences between the thoughts of people with OCD and these 'normal' intrusive thoughts. The intrusive thoughts that people who did not have OCD (or other problems) disclosed concerned impulses to hurt and abuse others, images of harm and thoughts that things were wrong or could go wrong. The content of the thoughts that others just had very fleetingly was remarkably similar to the thoughts that troubled people with OCD. The fact that 'normal' people experience all sorts of negative 'intrusive thoughts' is a very important fact to remember.

## THE NATURE OF THOUGHTS

Although we now know that negative and unacceptable intrusive thoughts are normal, clearly some people are much more troubled by them than others. Some people are so disturbed by their intrusive thoughts that, understandably, they would like to stop thinking them altogether. If only there was a way not to think about things being contaminated, or to block out the horrific and unwanted thoughts of violence, then surely the problem would be solved? This might seem like an attractive idea, but is it a realistic solution? What happens if you try? It has been known for many years now that the harder you try to get rid of an idea the more you will be troubled by it ... until you stop trying! As discussed later in this book, this is an example of *the solution becoming the problem*. The harder you try to get rid of your thoughts, the more important you are making them seem and the deeper the 'groove' they wear in your thinking patterns.

The reason you can't control your intrusive thoughts in this way is probably because you are not meant to! Our brain is designed as a super-efficient problem-solving machine which is flexible enough to adapt to unexpected situations. A really important thing in unexpected situations is to be able to free your thinking to come up with loads of different ways of tackling things, and to do that quickly. Probably for that reason, our brains tend to interrupt what we are doing with multiple ideas that *might be* relevant to what's going on. That's what intrusive thoughts are; a mishmash of things which spring to mind, especially when we are in an emotional (that is, important) situation. When it seems like we are in danger, our quick-fire mind gives us as many options as possible ... run away, climb a tree, fight, do nothing and so on. A lot of the options are irrelevant, stupid and dangerous, but the point is that our mind delivers as many of these as possible as quickly as possible. It is then up to the rational bit of us to choose which option to go for. What this means is that *we can't control intrusive thoughts*, but it is entirely within our control to respond or not respond to them as we think best. The ones we *do things about* will tend to stick around and are more likely to come back later. Unfortunately, this might include the thoughts we struggled to get rid of, or that we acted on defensively (for example by checking, washing our hands, or avoiding something). So attempts to defend ourselves against the intrusions keep us worried about them.

What this means is that if you could control some thoughts, you would have to do it by controlling all of your thoughts, to ensure that this was going to be effective. Funnily enough, this might have already happened in a particularly nasty way if you have OCD. Because the obsessions (and fighting them) have taken up so much of your attention, you may not have spent much time considering and noticing the other thoughts you have. Also, you may have given up thinking about some of the better things that might otherwise have been running round your head. So think back over the last few hours, or if you have just woken up, over the previous day. What kinds of thoughts have been going through your mind? Perhaps you had some thoughts about boring, tedious things you had to do, like the washing-up, or remembering to pay a bill? Did you have some positive thoughts about something nice you did in the past, or something you were looking forward to? Did you worry about anything, or did something upset you? Most likely you had thoughts in all of these categories. The point is that we have thoughts and images going through our mind much of the time. Sometimes, and in fact most of the time, thoughts such as these just 'pop' into our mind without us being aware of any 'chain of thought'. We might have a brilliant creative idea in this way, or suddenly remember to our horror that it was our turn to pick the children up from school an hour ago! This sort of 'intrusive' thought can be very useful indeed. Usually people can think of an occasion when they suddenly had a thought that was helpful, such as remembering a friend's birthday is coming up, or having a memory of a lovely holiday pop into their head.

Our everyday intrusive thoughts are generally not linear, ordered or controlled and that is a very good thing. Imagine what life would be like if they were and we had to plan everything we thought (if that was possible). There would be no creativity, no inspiration and no doing things on the spur of the moment and it would be a strange, dull and inhuman world. What this really means is that getting rid of the thoughts isn't a realistic, or even desirable, goal. Thoughts come and go, and are as important as we make them. Think of it as like a huge self-service cafeteria you are walking through with a tray. So many different things come to your attention. Oh yuk! There is the food which makes you sick. Would it be a good idea to focus on how much you don't want to take it? Or should you just accept that it's there and see what else is on offer? If you do, you can take that and tuck into your preferred choice. Pretty soon, the nasty smell will have faded from memory and you can carry on dealing with what you want, rather than being preoccupied with something which you can't stand.

> **KEY IDEA**
>
> So we know that 'intrusive thoughts' are entirely normal and may actually be helpful. Therefore having the thoughts themselves is **not** the problem. Simply stopping thinking the thoughts is an impossible goal.

So, if it is 'normal' and common to experience thoughts which are both unbidden and negative we need to look a bit further to understand why, for some people, having these thoughts is particularly worrying.

## THE 'COGNITIVE THEORY' OF EMOTION AND EMOTIONAL PROBLEMS

Cognitive theories and cognitive therapy were devised by Professor Aaron 'Tim' Beck, originally a psychoanalyst, who found he was bothered by two things as he tried to make the theories devised by Sigmund Freud work. Firstly, it seemed to Beck that psychoanalysis did not work when it was used to try to help patients. Secondly, the theory of emotions that psychoanalysis laid out also did not work when it was researched properly. At first Beck just found this confusing, but subsequently he used his findings to develop a cognitive theory of emotion and emotional disorders. He went on to apply this more specifically to develop a cognitive theory of depression, which provided the cornerstone for subsequent work in the cognitive understanding of many other problems, and the treatments that have proved so successful.

'Cognition' is another word for thoughts and meanings, so the cognitive theory was a theory of the role that thinking plays in a problem. In summary, Beck's theory stated that people did not become upset, anxious, sad or angry because of what happened to them, but instead by what they thought it meant (the way in which they interpreted it).

For example, imagine you were alone in the house and woke up in the middle of the night thinking you had heard a noise in the next room. If you thought it was an intruder, you would probably be frightened. However, when you then heard another noise ('miaow!') you would feel much better because you realised that it was not an intruder but your cat. This very simple example illustrates not only the way that negative thinking can make us needlessly anxious, but also the fact that changing our thinking (by finding out what is *really* happening in a particular situation) can help us feel quite differently.

So, Tim Beck showed us that depression was not caused directly by what happened to people, but by the interpretation given to those events. Furthermore, he suggested that how people saw and interpreted what happened to them was connected to their beliefs about themselves, about the world in general and also their beliefs about the future. People tend to think in a particular way because of past experiences which influenced what they believed about themselves and the world. For example, someone may have learned that 'the world is a dangerous place and you should trust no one'. Although this belief might seem to keep them safe, it would also have the effect of making them overly cautious and distrustful. The theory also suggests that this kind of belief can have the effect of changing the way the person experiences things. For example, it might result in the person being on the lookout for bad things happening and people not being trustworthy, so they did not notice when good things happened and people were helpful and reliable.

Thus, this theory went a long way in explaining why certain events affect some people more than others. For example, a person who has lost their job (the event) interprets it as 'I'm useless and inadequate and will never be able to keep a job'. This not only makes them feel sad, but means that they stop trying to get another job and withdraw to bed for days on end. However, another person may think 'This job didn't suit me; this is an opportunity to try something new'. They may feel slightly sad and a bit apprehensive about what a new job might be like (and how easy it would be to get one) but they would feel motivated to set in motion what they need to do in order to get a new job.

The same thing has happened to them, but these two people feel and behave very differently. The important point is that the response to any event hinges on the particular appraisal or meaning given to it by an individual.

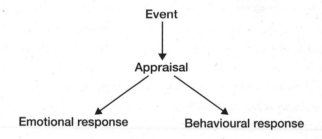

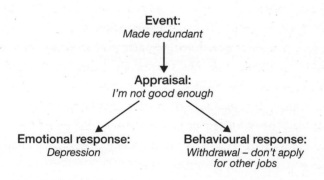

Let's consider some further examples when the appraisal of an event affects what emotion someone feels and what they do.

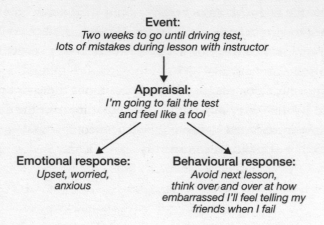

**Event:**
*Two weeks to go until driving test,
lots of mistakes during lesson with instructor*

**Appraisal:**
*I'm going to fail the test
and feel like a fool*

**Emotional response:**
*Upset, worried,
anxious*

**Behavioural response:**
*Avoid next lesson,
think over and over at how
embarrassed I'll feel telling my
friends when I fail*

By avoiding the lesson, they actually increase their chances of failing – a counterproductive course of action.

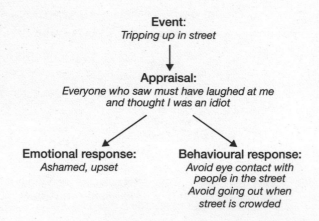

**Event:**
*Tripping up in street*

**Appraisal:**
*Everyone who saw must have laughed at me
and thought I was an idiot*

**Emotional response:**
*Ashamed, upset*

**Behavioural response:**
*Avoid eye contact with
people in the street
Avoid going out when
street is crowded*

By withdrawing, the person does not get the chance to find out what really happens when you trip in the street – that people either don't notice, or are sympathetic.

When this theory is applied to OCD, the event in question is not something in the outside world, but it is the mental event, i.e. the intrusive thought/urge/doubt/image or impulse itself. We know that intrusive thoughts are normal and very common, so the difference between someone who is bothered by a thought and someone who is not lies in *what they make* of having the thought. This 'appraisal' is what the intrusive thought seems to them to mean, for example, 'Having this thought means that I am a bad person'. It is important to note that it is not the case that negative intrusive thoughts never bother people who do not have OCD. For example, having an image of someone you love coming to harm, or a doubt as to whether you turned off the oven, would be experienced as uncomfortable to some extent for the majority of people. However, most people would consider these to be 'just one of those odd thoughts' and they would not spend any time thinking about why they had this thought, or consider having it as an urgent sign that they must act to undo or prevent harm. When a person has OCD, *having the thought itself* is often interpreted as being particularly significant and it is this significance which both drives the emotional response (such as anxiety, shame, misery) and motivates the need to do something about it (behavioural response).

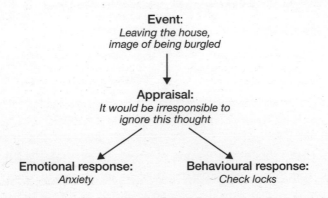

**Event:**
*Leaving the house,*
*image of being burgled*

**Appraisal:**
*It would be irresponsible to*
*ignore this thought*

**Emotional response:**
*Anxiety*

**Behavioural response:**
*Check locks*

Using our examples of intrusive thoughts, possible appraisals that could lead to significant anxiety are given below.

| INTRUSIVE THOUGHT | POSSIBLE APPRAISAL |
|---|---|
| **Thought** | |
| 'There might be blood in my food' | I could catch a disease and die |
| 'That is contaminated with germs' | I might be responsible for spreading contamination |
| 'My appointment is on Friday 13th' | Something bad might happen if I go |
| 'Have I left the front door open?' | Someone could break in and steal everything and it would be my fault |
| 'Did I run someone over without realising it?' | I could be a killer |
| **Images** | |
| Mum dead in a car crash | This could be a premonition |
| Abusing a baby or child | Having this thought must mean that I am a monster |
| **Urges** | |
| 'I must touch that or I won't feel right' | I could feel uncomfortable for ever |
| To jump in front of a train | I might be crazy |
| To physically assault someone | I am capable of doing something terrible |

These are, of course, just examples; sometimes the meaning of a person's thought is unique to them. In general, the meaning always concerns something negative or unsafe about the person themselves or the world in general and it is this which causes such anxiety. The meaning is also linked to the person's values, and significance is given to thoughts which appear to contradict them. For example, the gentle person who has violent thoughts would find these more upsetting than the thug, and the religious person experiencing blasphemous thoughts would find these much more problematic than an atheist. We will discuss this further in Chapter 2.

---

**KEY IDEA**

It is the personal meaning of the thoughts that makes them so unpleasant, anxiety-provoking and difficult to dismiss.

---

## COMPULSIONS

Compulsions (also called neutralising or safety-seeking behaviours) are the physical or mental actions and reactions that follow from intrusive thoughts or obsessions, and which are motivated by the meaning which the intrusion has for them. There are two main types of compulsions, which are best understood in terms of what the person is trying to do. One is to *verify* (to check, to make sure of) something, most commonly by physical or mental checking. The idea is that if you verify things, you can either feel completely sure that it is okay, or put it right if it is not. The second type of compulsion, *restitution*, is where the person aims to put right, make amends or correct something they think has already happened, for example by cleaning something thoroughly which they regard as contaminated, or by thinking a positive thought after having a negative thought they regard as dangerous.

People typically carry out compulsions for two important reasons: firstly, to try to prevent the harm for which they fear they might be responsible from happening, and secondly to reduce their levels of discomfort (anxiety, shame, sadness, anger). As such, the compulsions make sense as a response motivated by how a person has interpreted the obsessions. For example, if you are very worried about making yourself or others ill by contaminating them with something you have on your hands or body, it makes sense to do a lot of cleaning and washing. If you feel anxious that something may happen to a loved one, you do everything you can to make sure it doesn't happen. In addition to the (sometimes, but not always) anxiety-reducing effect of that, you may have found that going through a ritual relieves or soothes this anxiety for a short time, sometimes by taking your mind away from the main worry. Although it is understandable why people suffering from OCD do rituals in this way (including seeking reassurance from others), in the longer term the effect is to increase worry, preoccupation and anxiety. It is a bit like using a drug; it may make you feel better immediately, but you pay for your relief in the longer term by needing to ritualise and avoid more and more.

Compulsions at their most obvious can be physical actions which would be visible to someone else present (known as overt compulsions) or behaviours that go on in your own head (known as covert compulsions), such as checking your memory, saying a prayer or 'good word' after thinking something 'bad', and even internally arguing with oneself. It is also possible, and very common, to undertake more than one compulsion in response to a particular obsessional thought. There are also a number of other possible reactions to having obsessions such as avoidance of particular people, places or activities or trying to push the thoughts away (these will be discussed in much more detail later). Common compulsions and the obsessions and appraisals that they are often related to are shown below.

| INTRUSIVE THOUGHT | POSSIBLE APPRAISAL | COMPULSION |
|---|---|---|
| **Thought** | | |
| 'There might be blood in my food' | I could catch a disease and die | Check all food carefully |
| 'That is contaminated with germs' | I might be responsible for spreading contamination | Wash self and home |
| 'My appointment is on Friday 13th' | Something bad might happen if I go | Change the appointment |
| 'Have I left the front door open?' | Someone could break in and steal everything and it would be my fault | Go back and check |
| 'Did I run someone over without realising it?' | I could be a killer | Go back and check; listen out for unusual noises when driving |
| **Images** | | |
| Mum dead in a car crash | This could be a premonition | Cross fingers and think of a positive image |
| Abusing a baby or child | I must be a paedophile | Avoid all children |
| **Urges** | | |
| 'I must touch that or I won't feel right' | I could feel uncomfortable for ever | Touch it in groups of seven until feeling goes |
| To jump in front of a train | I might be crazy | Never go near platform edge |
| To physically assault someone | I am capable of doing something terrible | Sit on hands |

# IMPAIRMENT AND DISTRESS

The final element in understanding OCD is the interference caused by the problem. Interference seems too mild a word for the havoc wreaked by this problem. The negative appraisals in OCD invariably cause anxiety (often escalating into sheer terror) but can also be linked with other negative emotions such as shame, depression, disgust and anger. The anxiety is significant, that is, it tends to last for a long time and comes back after a short while. Continuously or repeatedly feeling anxious is very unpleasant in itself. Feeling unsafe and anxious can also affect your sleep and appetite and can cause you to become irritable with those around you. If you perform compulsions to try to manage these feelings or to stop bad things happening, it is likely that the urge to do this does not always come at a 'convenient' time. Most people with OCD find that they begin to prioritise their rituals and compulsions over other things and may find that doing compulsions takes up increasing amounts of time. This then has a knock-on effect on other things. Often this means being late for activities and appointments, or avoiding particular places or situations to try to avoid the stress and anxiety from having negative thoughts or doing compulsions. You may be missing out on certain social activities, or may avoid taking on more challenging jobs due to obsessions and compulsions. People can spend vast amounts of money they can't afford on cleaning and washing products or getting rid of things that seem to them marred, spoiled or contaminated. Sometimes people go to great lengths, even moving house or country to try to get away from 'contamination'.

Friends and families are often very concerned about a loved one who is caught up in rituals and obsessions. It can be heartbreaking to see someone in states of high distress, and it may be very difficult for you to explain what is happening if you are not sure yourself or if you are experiencing a great deal of shame about your difficulties. If you are doing a lot of compulsions such as cleaning, it may be difficult for those who live with you to follow the same rules or live up to the same standards as, if they do not have an obsessional problem, they probably do not share the same underlying beliefs or concerns. Following your rules may be stressful for you and for them, and this issue often causes conflicts within families. We will talk more about this and how to tackle it in Chapter 8.

Although some people with obsessive–compulsive disorder are able to continue to work and have a social life, others find that they have no choice but to give up most other things, de facto becoming full-time OCDers. OCD tends to creep into more and more areas of your life, taking it over.

---

**KEY IDEA**

Compulsions make sense as a response to the interpretation of obsessions. However, they are likely to have an increasingly negative impact on you and those around you.

---

## SELF-ASSESSMENT SECTION: SO DO I HAVE OCD?

Below are some of the symptoms people commonly experience as part of OCD. As you will see, the items describe thoughts and behaviours in a quite general way. This is because the specific content of worries and particular behaviours can be very individual. The questionnaire asks you to think about how much distress the particular symptom is causing you. There is no particular number that indicates whether you have OCD, as some people will be bothered by many of the things listed below, while others will be bothered by only a few. The purpose of the questionnaire is to get you thinking not just about whether you have obsessions or compulsions but about the degree to which you are *bothered* by these types of symptoms. This is a questionnaire that has been used extensively in clinical work and research. Try not to worry if you don't understand every statement or you think it doesn't apply to you – just move on to the next item.

## OBSESSIVE–COMPULSIVE INVENTORY

The following statements refer to experiences which many people have in their everyday lives. In the column labelled DISTRESS, please circle the number that best describes how much that experience has distressed or bothered you during the past month. The numbers in this column refer to the following labels:

**DISTRESS**

0 = Not at all   1 = A little   2 = Moderately   3 = A lot   4 = Extremely

1.  Unpleasant thoughts come into my mind against my will and I cannot get rid of them.          0   1   2   3   4

2.  I think contact with bodily secretions (perspiration, saliva, blood, urine, etc) may contaminate my clothes or somehow harm me.          0   1   2   3   4

3.  I ask people to repeat things to me several times, even though I understood them the first time.          0   1   2   3   4

4.  I wash and clean obsessively.          0   1   2   3   4

5.  I have to review mentally past events, conversations and actions to make sure that I didn't do something wrong.

          0   1   2   3   4

6.  I have saved up so many things that they get in the way.

          0   1   2   3   4

7.  I check things more often than necessary.          0   1   2   3   4

8.  I avoid using public toilets because I am afraid of disease or contamination.          0   1   2   3   4

9.  I repeatedly check doors, windows, drawers, etc.

          0   1   2   3   4

10. I repeatedly check gas and water taps and light switches after turning them off.       0 1 2 3 4

11. I collect things I don't need.       0 1 2 3 4

12. I have thoughts of having hurt someone without knowing it.       0 1 2 3 4

13. I have thoughts that I might want to harm myself or others.       0 1 2 3 4

14. I get upset if objects are not arranged properly.       0 1 2 3 4

15. I feel obliged to follow a particular order in dressing, undressing and washing myself.       0 1 2 3 4

16. I feel compelled to count while I am doing things.       0 1 2 3 4

17. I am afraid of impulsively doing embarrassing or harmful things.       0 1 2 3 4

18. I need to pray to cancel bad thoughts or feelings.       0 1 2 3 4

19. I keep on checking forms or other things I have written.       0 1 2 3 4

20. I get upset at the sight of knives, scissors and other sharp objects in case I lose control with them.       0 1 2 3 4

21. I am excessively concerned about cleanliness. 0 1 2 3 4

22. I find it difficult to touch an object when I know it has been touched by strangers or certain people.       0 1 2 3 4

23. I need things to be arranged in a particular order.       0 1 2 3 4

24. I get behind in my work because I repeat things over and over again.       0 1 2 3 4

25. I feel I have to repeat certain numbers.       0 1 2 3 4

26. After doing something carefully, I still have the impression I have not finished it.       0 1 2 3 4

27. I find it difficult to touch garbage or dirty things.       0 1 2 3 4

28. I find it difficult to control my own thoughts.       0 1 2 3 4

29. I have to do things over and over again until it feels right.       0 1 2 3 4

30. I am upset by unpleasant thoughts that come into my mind against my will.       0 1 2 3 4

31. Before going to sleep I have to do certain things in a certain way.       0 1 2 3 4

32. I go back to places to make sure that I have not harmed anyone.       0 1 2 3 4

33. I frequently get nasty thoughts and have difficulty in getting rid of them.       0 1 2 3 4

34. I avoid throwing things away because I am afraid I might need them later.       0 1 2 3 4

35. I get upset if others change the way I have arranged my things.       0 1 2 3 4

36. I feel that I must repeat certain words or phrases in my mind in order to wipe out bad thoughts, feelings or actions.       0 1 2 3 4

37. After I have done things, I have persistent doubts about whether I really did them.       0 1 2 3 4

38. I sometimes have to wash or clean myself simply because I feel contaminated.       0 1 2 3 4

39. I feel that there are good and bad numbers. 0 1 2 3 4

40. I repeatedly check anything which might cause a fire.       0 1 2 3 4

41. Even when I do something very carefully I feel that it is not quite right.                                     0  1  2  3  4

42. I wash my hands more often or longer than necessary.
                                     0  1  2  3  4

Foa E., Kozak M., Salkovskis, P., Coles M., Amir N. (1998), 'The validation of a new obsessive-compulsive disorder scale: The Obsessive-Compulsive Inventory', *Psychological Assessment*, 10(3), 206–214.

## MY PROBLEM DOESN'T FIT: I DON'T HAVE COMPULSIONS

Sometimes people are acutely aware that they have unpleasant obsessional thoughts, but do not feel that they have any compulsions. This may be the case, and you may be continuing your life despite having lots of obsessions. Sometimes people say that although they are not performing obvious compulsions in terms of what they do, the quality of their life is affected by the torment caused by their obsessions. Compulsions are in fact always there, but they can be hidden. In some cases the compulsions are very subtle and may be more related to avoiding particular activities. In others the compulsions are all internal (often referred to as 'neutralising'), including not only mental checking by going over things in your mind and restitution in which you try to 'put things right' in your head (by thinking a good thought to balance a bad one, for example) but also things like mental arguing (trying to convince yourself that there is nothing to worry about, a type of self-reassurance seeking) or by directly seeking reassurance from those around you. Whether your compulsions are external, like washing or checking, or internal, like neutralising, it is still obsessive–compulsive disorder.

## MY PROBLEM DOESN'T FIT: I DON'T HAVE OBSESSIONS

It is also the case that people find it hard to describe the particular thoughts related to their compulsions. For example, if you are very used to washing your hands in a ritualistic manner, then you may do this each time whether or not you have a particular thought. However, it is likely that when it originally developed, the behaviour was a response to a thought and has, with the passage of time, become more like a habit that is done automatically. One way of thinking about this is if you drive a car (or if not, when crossing the road as a pedestrian), you probably stop at red traffic lights quite habitually. How often do you think about why you stop, or the consequences of not stopping when you approach a red light? Most people do not think about it at all, but of course the reason you do stop is to avoid an accident when cars or people are crossing the road ahead of you. If your brakes were to fail when you were approaching a red light, the underlying reasons for stopping will come flooding back quickly and vividly!

For those people with no obvious obsessional thought, the fact that you are continuing to do your rituals or compulsions, even though there is a cost to you in terms of time taken up, interference with your life and distress, suggests that there is an underlying reason that is preventing you just giving them up, and that underlying reason will be a submerged and invisible obsessional thought which you have stopped being aware of, in the same way that you have stopped being aware of why you stop at a red traffic light. The only way to find out what this is is to conduct your own 'experiment', where you actively try to stop doing the ritual or compulsion. This is, of course, very hard to do, and it might be a good idea to seek support from someone close to you when you try to do it. This also has the advantage of giving you someone to talk to about it when you have tried this experiment. Some people reading this book might not have told anyone at all about their problem. Although understandable, perhaps this is now the time to open up to someone you trust, so that you can get the support that you need to help you change.

Usually the obsessional thoughts related to the compulsions come to the forefront of a person's mind when they do this 'finding out' exercise (i.e. when you try to actively stop doing the compulsion). You might also consider whether what is going on is happening as a mental image (a picture), impulse or urge, or a doubt about something you consider important. However, this is not always the case and you should not worry if it is hard to identify clear obsessional thoughts. For a small number of people, the obsessional thoughts have faded away to nothing, leaving the compulsion as a habit. If this is the case, then you can simply phase out the compulsion.

## HOW ARE OBSESSIONS AND COMPULSIONS AFFECTING YOU?

When it takes hold, OCD can affect many areas in a person's life. However, it doesn't always start like that. For some, the OCD takes the disguise of a friend, promising to keep you safe … but at a very high cost! And as time goes on, that cost escalates and keeps on rising. It can affect your well-being in a general way if you are constantly feeling anxious and can also have a direct impact on what you feel you can do and where you feel you can go. In many cases it can have an impact on relationships with other people, as they are repeatedly asked for reassurance or won't follow your obsessional rules. It is worth asking yourself what is the real cost of your problem. Do the obsessions or compulsions take a lot of your time? Do they get in the way of your plans to do other things? Have family members complained? Are you frequently late? Are you suffering from physical problems such as rashes or dry skin? Are you spending a lot of money on replacing contaminated things or buying cleaning products? Perhaps you have decided not to take on a more challenging role or course, as these would be hard to manage around your obsessions or compulsions. You may even have decided not to have a relationship or not to have children due to fears and worries related to OCD.

Think about all of these areas and note whether and how the problem is affecting each one:

- Time
- Money
- Ability to have emotional and physical intimacy
- Family members and friends
- Job/education

If the descriptions of obsessions and compulsions fit with things that you are thinking and doing, it is possible that you may have OCD at some level. The clinical diagnosis of OCD is given when people have either obsessions or compulsions that significantly interfere with their lives, and it is the level of interference which is key. Usually this means that people are particularly troubled, or are spending a lot of time on their obsessions and compulsions. However, many people have symptoms of OCD at a lower level which can still cause some interference and inconvenience. The symptoms may increase if their circumstances change and they experience more stresses in their lives. We know that many people coming to treatment wait for a long time until things get really bad before seeking help, with one study identifying an average wait of 11 years. Understanding the nature of OCD can help prevent the problem growing and as you will see, you can use the techniques in this book even if you have low levels of the problem or if you have recovered

If OCD is causing significant interference in your life it is important to acknowledge this reality. Even if this is difficult, it is the springboard for thinking about why it's so important to change, and for imagining how you would like your life to be without this problem. We will return to this at the end of Chapter 3 when we ask you to identify your goals.

# HOW DO YOU KNOW IF YOUR FRIEND OR FAMILY MEMBER HAS OCD?

You may be reading this book because you are concerned about a friend or family member and suspect that their behaviour could mean that they have OCD. It is often the case that family and friends are aware of the anxiety, distress and impairment caused by the problem, even if the particular obsessions and compulsions are well hidden. There are many different types of OCD, and some fears and compulsions are much more apparent than others to an observer. Friends and family may notice somebody checking a lock repeatedly, washing something excessively or repeating a physical activity. Less obvious are mental rituals like replacing 'bad' thoughts with 'good' ones, saying a silent prayer or self-reassurance. You may have noticed your friend or family member being very quiet in certain situations, or saying something under their breath. However, there are many compulsions and reactions driven by OCD that can be going on in the person's mind without anyone else knowing.

Another, very important, issue is that due to the shame and secrecy that often surrounds OCD, people can become very good at hiding their symptoms, or delaying their rituals until they are alone. People with OCD can become very skilled at generating subtle excuses so they can avoid situations where their problem will be worse. The general stigma of 'mental health' problems may also stop people from talking about their difficulties. It is useful to remember that, for these reasons, OCD can sometimes be difficult to spot. However, if OCD is around, you have probably noticed its effects, even if they are subtle.

In the table below we give a range of examples of what family and friends may notice in the behaviour of a loved one and how it might be related to certain forms of OCD. By reading further into this book it will become clear how and why each one of these can result from obsessional fears.

| WHAT FAMILY AND FRIENDS MAY NOTICE | EXAMPLES OF FORMS OF OCD THAT OFTEN RESULT IN THIS BEHAVIOUR |
| --- | --- |
| They are frequently late | Various forms of OCD that involve lengthy checking/washing/other rituals |
| They find it very difficult to delegate tasks that might involve 'risk', e.g. locking the back door OR delegate ALL such tasks to another person | Various forms of OCD; often checking OCD |
| They find everyday tasks (e.g. driving, cooking dinner) very difficult or delegate them for unknown reasons | Various forms of OCD, for example a fear of accidentally poisoning someone leading to avoidance of cooking |
| They ask you for reassurance regularly | Potentially all forms of OCD; an explicit example would be asking for reassurance that a door is shut (checking OCD); a more subtle example would be frequent phone calls to check that you are okay (OCD related to feeling an inflated sense of responsibility for your safety) |
| They are anxious, irritable or angry if you interrupt their routine or break their rules | Potentially all forms of OCD; an example would be someone with extensive washing rituals that are carried out in a certain order to avoid 'contamination' from one body part to the next – to interrupt or interfere in this ritual would mean that they would 'lose track' of contamination and would have to start the lengthy process again |

| WHAT FAMILY AND FRIENDS MAY NOTICE | EXAMPLES OF FORMS OF OCD THAT OFTEN RESULT IN THIS BEHAVIOUR |
| --- | --- |
| They avoid particular places or being with particular people or categories of people (e.g. children, the elderly) | Potentially all forms of OCD; for example, someone with intrusive thoughts of harm towards vulnerable people |
| They repeat routine activities trying to get them exactly right or 'perfect' (e.g. writing an email or letter) | Various forms of OCD including where things need to 'feel right' |
| They ask you to follow particular rules that don't seem to make sense or be necessary (e.g. everyone has to change their clothes when they come into the house) | Often contamination OCD, but can be other forms of OCD |
| The person spends a long time washing their hands, bathing and/or cleaning | Usually contamination OCD |
| Their skin is red and dry, particularly on their hands | Usually contamination OCD |
| The washing machine is constantly on/ the house always smells strongly of cleaning products | Usually contamination, but can be other forms of OCD |
| They often want to, or do spend money on replacing things which do not need replacing | Usually contamination OCD |
| They spend a long time leaving the house | Usually checking OCD |
| They are very distant and preoccupied | Rumination and religious OCD but can be others |

If the person you are concerned about is not sure if they have OCD you can go through this book together to see if these are the sorts of things that are happening and whether the understanding of OCD we talk about in the next chapters fits with what they are experiencing. There is some information on page 233 about other problems which can seem similar to OCD and how to get help for them.

## WHEN THE PERSON YOU ARE WORRIED ABOUT IS RELUCTANT TO TALK ABOUT IT

Sometimes friends and family members may open the discussion before the person themselves, and sometimes things get to such a point that they feel forced to do so. There are two main reasons that people may not recognise the problem or seek help in the early stages. For some people, OCD can *seem* like a helpful friend at first as it may give them a sense of control in difficult circumstances. What can start as 'normal behaviours' can then gradually become excessive and harmful. Others may be very afraid of what is going through their mind and have no other way to make sense of it than that they are bad, mad or dangerous. This horrible fear may stop them disclosing the problem to anyone, even those they love, for fear of the consequences.

## TRY TO BRING IT UP

It is always worth trying to discuss the problem with the person you are worried about, even in general terms – after all, you are asking because you have noticed something is up, even if they are trying to hide it. Sometimes being asked what's wrong can be a great relief as things get into the open and they no longer have to cover it up, or worry about your reaction. If they have not yet discussed it then it may be because they feel very ashamed of their thoughts and behaviour and it may be difficult to go into detail. Assure them that you don't need to know all the details if they don't want to tell you but you just want to help them with an obviously distressing problem. Alternatively, they may feel embarrassed or 'silly' talking about the things they are doing (but this is replaced by real fear or anxiety when they are stuck in their obsessions and compulsions). Using some of the examples in this book might help your friend or family member to realise that they are not alone.

## BEING SENSITIVE

It goes without saying that it is important to try to be as sensitive and understanding as possible and let people tell you in their own way, and in their own time. Some people like very 'matter-of-fact' conversations, some people might prefer an email, some people might like the analogies and metaphors we have used in this book as an opening to a conversation. Your friend or family member may feel more comfortable discussing their problems if they know about something you have struggled with in *your* life. The most important thing is letting them know that you want to help *them* work out what is happening, as this is the way they will overcome the problem. There is more information aimed at helping friends and family support someone fighting the problem in Chapter 8.

## QUESTIONS YOU MIGHT ASK SOMEONE YOU THINK MAY HAVE OCD

- I've seen you are often quite anxious (when you are leaving the house/preparing food/walking in a certain street/around children, etc). What are you worrying about when you feel that way?
- I've noticed that you (wash/check) quite a lot, more than most people. How much are you doing that/how much time are you spending? Do *you* think what you are doing is excessive?
- Sometimes people worry about the thoughts they have and this can be part of a problem called OCD – is that something you are worrying about?

# 2

# HOW DID I DEVELOP OCD?

Now you have an understanding of the different elements of OCD and the importance of *meaning* in driving the problem.

This chapter will build on this to help you think about:

- *Why* different people may have different meanings
- Other factors important in developing OCD, including:
  - biological factors
  - psychological factors
  - external events

The first chapter should have given you a clear idea of what are obsessions and compulsions and how to recognise them. It should also have begun to make sense of why obsessional thoughts cause so much anxiety and why people feel strongly compelled to perform compulsions, i.e. the central meaning given to the thoughts. The meaning is usually that having a particular thought:

1. Means something bad about you related to what you are doing or thinking, and/or
2. That something bad might happen because of what you do (or don't do) and that therefore you should, and indeed must, act because of this sense of responsibility.

We know that not everyone responds to their thoughts in this way and that, for many people, even the most violent and chilling thoughts can be easily ignored *because they don't carry the burden of meaning*. This means that those who don't have OCD typically treat their intrusive thoughts, images and doubts as mostly irrelevant. As a result, they do not respond in the ways which typically tend to keep OCD in place; that is, they don't use compulsive behaviour, avoidance, thought suppression and all the other things motivated by fears of being responsible for harm. To continue the task of really getting inside this problem, this chapter will cover the reasons that some people may be more susceptible to such fears of being responsible for harm and therefore the negative interpretations of thoughts associated with OCD.

## NO SIMPLE ANSWERS: THE VULNERABILITY–STRESS MODEL

Where do mental health problems come from? Put simply, it is reasonable to say that people experience psychological problems because things get to them in ways that they can't manage and through no fault of their own. This simple truth can conceal another, as researchers ignore the complexity of human beings and their problems and try to pin down blame for problems such as OCD to genes, brain chemical imbalances or a troubled relationship with parents. Appealing though such simple explanations are, the less obvious truth is that the causes of psychological problems are complex and interlinked. There appear to be several different ways in which a person can end up suffering from a problem such as OCD and it is never simple.

Everybody has a combination of vulnerabilities and strengths ('resilience'). Research and experience tells us that there are many types of biological, environmental and psychological factors that might be linked to why a person develops mental health problems. However, there are also things which can protect us from even the most severe circumstances. In other words, we all have our limits, and if pushed far enough anyone can and will experience severe and persistent mental health problems. How far we have to be pushed before 'breaking down', and the way in which such a 'breakdown' will affect us, will depend on several of these factors, some general, for example, how mentally 'tough' we are, how we seek support from those around us (or don't), some specific, for example, our weak spots ('Achilles heel'), our ways of coping when confronted by problems. And, of course, this will also relate to the type of pressure we find ourselves under and our past experience of such problems and dealing with them.

To complicate things further, some of these factors are thought to represent very general vulnerabilities to stress (such as how easily we become worried and how we physically react to stressful situations), while others may present specific risks linked to a particular problem, such as our sensitivity to particular types of worries. It goes on to become even more complicated; these factors will also vary depending on day-to-day issues, such as whether we are feeling run down, our reactions to recent events (such as bereavements, falling in love), our mood, having had too much coffee and feeling on edge and so on. Notice that these factors can go either way, making you more or less susceptible to problems. And of course, the reality is that there is always a complicated combination of factors involved in complicated ways. Happy events can increase our fears. For example, having a baby can, for most people, open up whole new worlds of joy and opportunity, but can also unleash a world of uncertainty and terror about things which can go wrong. For someone who is worried already, things going well becomes another source of worry, as the person realises how much they now have to lose!

This complicated pattern of factors has been described as the 'vulnerability–stress' model. The idea of a complicated interplay between how a person is 'made' and the things which happen to them is the accepted model of thinking about most physical and mental health problems. A combination of background factors including those related to genes, to social, psychological and biological factors and to past experience can make us more vulnerable to developing a problem in stressful circumstances. These factors may come into play in certain situations (such as external events), and the combination may then 'tip' us into the problem, which will be further affected by the way in which we try to 'fight it off' and the extent to which further events affect our ability to deal with the situation.

In reality, there is a lot of variation in the contribution of vulnerability and stress factors for individuals. It may be that one factor is particularly potent for one person, while for another it could be something completely different. The diagrams below illustrate this idea:

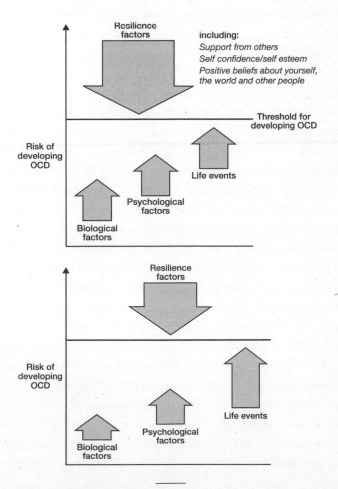

# BIOLOGICAL VULNERABILITIES

Are you a victim of your biology and genes? Some neuroscience researchers in the field of mental health have encouraged us to think of research on brain scans and similar findings as indicating that you are. This research is often described in terms of chemical imbalances in the brain, faulty brain circuitry, genetic defects and so on. However, people are often surprised to learn that the supposed genetic and other supposed vulnerabilities described in OCD are most likely to fall into the category of 'non-specific' risks for developing a disorder. An example of a non-specific risk would be the fact that women are twice as likely to be depressed as men. This does not mean, of course, that depression is caused by being a woman!

Yes, groups of people with OCD are sometimes found to have different patterns of brain activation when brain scans are carried out. However, it would be very weird if this were not true, given the way these studies are carried out. The brain scan is sensitive to different patterns of activity in the brain and can, for example, detect the difference in terms of the way the brain reacts between expert musicians listening to music and people with no special knowledge of music. It is therefore not surprising that there are brain activation differences between people with OCD and those without; they tend to have different patterns of worrying! This does not mean that OCD is a biological disease.

No true biological differences have been found between people with and without OCD, and those that have been identified are confused by the fact that having the disorder can lead to temporary changes in the brain, such as listening to music or thinking a happy thought. There is clearly no 'OCD gene', but certain genes have been implicated as vulnerability factors. These genes become relevant and 'switched on' in particular environments. This is true of all human behaviours, for example, having a genetic predisposition to being an amazing tree climber may not be relevant unless you live somewhere where you can climb trees regularly. We cannot do very much about the genetic hand which nature deals us, but we know that biology is only one aspect of vulnerability and that other factors (which can change) are necessary for a problem to develop. It is hard to estimate because the research findings are not clear, but probably less than 10% of what happens in OCD can be linked to genetic factors, and these factors are probably to do with being prone to anxiety; that is, 'being a bit of a worrier'.

---

**KEY IDEA**
At the time of writing, there is no biological theory of OCD which helps us understand it in ways which could improve how it is treated.

---

## PSYCHOLOGICAL VULNERABILITIES: THE SPECIAL ROLE OF RESPONSIBILITY

There is no doubt that OCD is a problem of thinking and how the sufferer reacts to their thoughts. We all have 'silent' beliefs about ourselves, how the world works, and our future; these are general attitudes which are based on our understanding of our place in the world, and are linked to the values by which we live our lives. These attitudes may not be something we are aware of most of the time and we may never even have thought much about them, but they are there and we act consistently with them. For example, if you are a person who has general attitudes about yourself that you are essentially good and competent, but one day your car breaks down and you lose your keys, you may think, 'what a lot of bad luck!' If you believe that you are in some way defective, you may conclude, 'bad things always happen to me'. Returning to Beck's cognitive model, he put forward the idea that the beliefs that a person holds about themselves and the world in general act like a lens through which they view what happens to them. They are the 'unwritten rules' of our life. It may be that specific events bring particular beliefs 'online' which were not previously relevant, for example, losing a job may bring to the front a person's belief that they are worthless. They may never have thought about this before, as things have generally gone okay for them; the unwritten rules were never challenged.

We build up our set of beliefs through a combination of direct experience and what we are told about ourselves and the world, over our entire life. It is therefore very difficult to pinpoint where beliefs come from, and in reality they are usually assembled and developed from many different sources over many years. A number of beliefs are relevant to the experience of OCD. These include the need to be 'perfect', the need to be 'in control' and difficulties in tolerating uncertainty. One set of beliefs that has been consistently shown to be very important in OCD is the set concerning responsibility for harm. This is the idea that by doing something wrong, or failing to act, you may be responsible for causing a terrible and preventable outcome. The 'terrible' thing may be very individual, and may involve harm coming to you or someone you love, or a complete stranger. The key factor is that by your actions (what you do or what you fail to do) you will be in some way to blame if it were to happen.

We know that people with OCD have very broad shoulders where responsibility is concerned; that is, they feel very aware of responsibility, and it is very hard for someone like that to tolerate the idea that they could be even partly responsible for something awful happening and not do something about it. As with other beliefs, these ideas build up over time, but theorists suggest that particular early experiences may play a role for some people. One example of this is being expected to, or made to, take on a lot of actual responsibility, perhaps by caring for siblings or even adults. Similarly, 'scapegoated' children who are consistently blamed by parents/carers for negative consequences over which they actually have little control (e.g. 'look what you've made me do now') may take on a broad sense of responsibility.

You may have had to follow very rigid and extreme codes of conduct and duty leading you to conclude that there are very bad moral consequences to certain actions. Some overly strict religious upbringings can have this effect; for OCD a highly relevant example is the idea of 'sin by thought'. See 'Superstition and magical thinking' on page 61. Everyday things, like the dangers of not being clean, can sow the seeds for obsessional fears about contamination and washing.

Alternatively, you may have been overprotected and shielded from ever taking responsibility, perhaps by being told that the world is too dangerous a place and that you are not able to operate successfully in it without taking a lot of care. When it is your turn to take responsibility this can therefore become particularly frightening, leading you to be so careful that you behave ... obsessionally.

---

**GENERAL BELIEFS COMMONLY ACCOMPANYING COMPULSIONS**
- If I don't act something bad will happen and it would be my fault
- Now I've thought of it, I should do something about it
- If I don't act I will feel very very anxious and it will never go away
- I have to be completely sure that I have not allowed something bad to happen

---

On occasion particular incidents happen in childhood that can lead to the development of beliefs around responsibility. This may be one specific incident or a series of incidents in which something you did or did not do actually contributed to a serious misfortune. Believing oneself to be inadvertently capable of causing something terrible to happen can lead people to believe it is their responsibility to take extra care. Sometimes, unfortunate coincidences can lead people to conclusions about their responsibility in misfortunes, perhaps thinking 'I wish you were dead' about someone who then died soon after. Through a number of different experiences, or sometimes one key experience, people with OCD have commonly absorbed the idea that it is very important that they take particular care about their thoughts and actions. This is a subtle type of responsibility belief, where your own thoughts can cause and/or prevent harm, making you responsible for it.

Below are some of the responsibility ideas that people commonly experience as part of OCD. The questionnaire asks you to think about how much you agree with the idea. There is no particular number of 'agrees' that indicates whether you have OCD; the purpose of the questionnaire is to get you thinking about whether you have inflated responsibility beliefs. This is a questionnaire that has been used extensively in clinical work and research. Try not to worry if you don't understand every statement or you think it doesn't apply to you – just move on to the next item.

---

**SELF ASSESSMENT: DO I HAVE INFLATED RESPONSIBILITY IDEAS?**

1. I often feel responsible for things which go wrong.

| TOTALLY AGREE | AGREE VERY MUCH | AGREE SLIGHTLY | NEUTRAL | DISAGREE SLIGHTLY | DISAGREE VERY MUCH | TOTALLY DISAGREE |
|---|---|---|---|---|---|---|

2. If I don't act when I can foresee danger, then I am to blame for any consequences if it happens.

| TOTALLY AGREE | AGREE VERY MUCH | AGREE SLIGHTLY | NEUTRAL | DISAGREE SLIGHTLY | DISAGREE VERY MUCH | TOTALLY DISAGREE |
|---|---|---|---|---|---|---|

3. I am too sensitive to feeling responsible for things going wrong.

| TOTALLY AGREE | AGREE VERY MUCH | AGREE SLIGHTLY | NEUTRAL | DISAGREE SLIGHTLY | DISAGREE VERY MUCH | TOTALLY DISAGREE |
|---|---|---|---|---|---|---|

---

4. If I think bad things, this is as bad as doing bad things.

| TOTALLY AGREE | AGREE VERY MUCH | AGREE SLIGHTLY | NEUTRAL | DISAGREE SLIGHTLY | DISAGREE VERY MUCH | TOTALLY DISAGREE |
|---|---|---|---|---|---|---|

5. I worry a great deal about the effects of things which I do or don't do.

| TOTALLY AGREE | AGREE VERY MUCH | AGREE SLIGHTLY | NEUTRAL | DISAGREE SLIGHTLY | DISAGREE VERY MUCH | TOTALLY DISAGREE |
|---|---|---|---|---|---|---|

6. To me, not acting to prevent disaster is as bad as making disaster happen.

| TOTALLY AGREE | AGREE VERY MUCH | AGREE SLIGHTLY | NEUTRAL | DISAGREE SLIGHTLY | DISAGREE VERY MUCH | TOTALLY DISAGREE |
|---|---|---|---|---|---|---|

7. If I know that harm is possible, I should always try to prevent it, however unlikely it seems.

| TOTALLY AGREE | AGREE VERY MUCH | AGREE SLIGHTLY | NEUTRAL | DISAGREE SLIGHTLY | DISAGREE VERY MUCH | TOTALLY DISAGREE |
|---|---|---|---|---|---|---|

8. I must always think through the consequences of even the smallest actions.

| TOTALLY AGREE | AGREE VERY MUCH | AGREE SLIGHTLY | NEUTRAL | DISAGREE SLIGHTLY | DISAGREE VERY MUCH | TOTALLY DISAGREE |
|---|---|---|---|---|---|---|

9. I often take responsibility for things which other people don't think are my fault.

| TOTALLY AGREE | AGREE VERY MUCH | AGREE SLIGHTLY | NEUTRAL | DISAGREE SLIGHTLY | DISAGREE VERY MUCH | TOTALLY DISAGREE |
|---|---|---|---|---|---|---|

10. Everything I do can cause serious problems.

| TOTALLY AGREE | AGREE VERY MUCH | AGREE SLIGHTLY | NEUTRAL | DISAGREE SLIGHTLY | DISAGREE VERY MUCH | TOTALLY DISAGREE |
|---|---|---|---|---|---|---|

11. I am often close to causing harm.

| TOTALLY AGREE | AGREE VERY MUCH | AGREE SLIGHTLY | NEUTRAL | DISAGREE SLIGHTLY | DISAGREE VERY MUCH | TOTALLY DISAGREE |
|---|---|---|---|---|---|---|

12. I must protect others from harm.

| TOTALLY AGREE | AGREE VERY MUCH | AGREE SLIGHTLY | NEUTRAL | DISAGREE SLIGHTLY | DISAGREE VERY MUCH | TOTALLY DISAGREE |
|---|---|---|---|---|---|---|

13. I should never cause even the slightest harm to others.

| TOTALLY AGREE | AGREE VERY MUCH | AGREE SLIGHTLY | NEUTRAL | DISAGREE SLIGHTLY | DISAGREE VERY MUCH | TOTALLY DISAGREE |
|---|---|---|---|---|---|---|

14. I will be condemned for my actions.

| TOTALLY AGREE | AGREE VERY MUCH | AGREE SLIGHTLY | NEUTRAL | DISAGREE SLIGHTLY | DISAGREE VERY MUCH | TOTALLY DISAGREE |
|---|---|---|---|---|---|---|

15. If I can have even a slight influence on things going wrong, then I must act to prevent it.

| TOTALLY AGREE | AGREE VERY MUCH | AGREE SLIGHTLY | NEUTRAL | DISAGREE SLIGHTLY | DISAGREE VERY MUCH | TOTALLY DISAGREE |
|---|---|---|---|---|---|---|

16. To me, not acting where disaster is a slight possibility is as bad as making that disaster happen.

| TOTALLY AGREE | AGREE VERY MUCH | AGREE SLIGHTLY | NEUTRAL | DISAGREE SLIGHTLY | DISAGREE VERY MUCH | TOTALLY DISAGREE |
|---|---|---|---|---|---|---|

17. For me, even slight carelessness is inexcusable when it might affect other people.

| TOTALLY AGREE | AGREE VERY MUCH | AGREE SLIGHTLY | NEUTRAL | DISAGREE SLIGHTLY | DISAGREE VERY MUCH | TOTALLY DISAGREE |
|---|---|---|---|---|---|---|

18. In all kinds of daily situations, my inactivity can cause as much harm as deliberate bad intentions.

| TOTALLY AGREE | AGREE VERY MUCH | AGREE SLIGHTLY | NEUTRAL | DISAGREE SLIGHTLY | DISAGREE VERY MUCH | TOTALLY DISAGREE |
|---|---|---|---|---|---|---|

19. Even if harm is a very unlikely possibility, I should always try to prevent it at any cost.

| TOTALLY AGREE | AGREE VERY MUCH | AGREE SLIGHTLY | NEUTRAL | DISAGREE SLIGHTLY | DISAGREE VERY MUCH | TOTALLY DISAGREE |
|---|---|---|---|---|---|---|

20. Once I think it is possible that I have caused harm, I can't forgive myself.

| TOTALLY AGREE | AGREE VERY MUCH | AGREE SLIGHTLY | NEUTRAL | DISAGREE SLIGHTLY | DISAGREE VERY MUCH | TOTALLY DISAGREE |
|---|---|---|---|---|---|---|

21. Many of my past actions have been intended to prevent harm to others.

| TOTALLY AGREE | AGREE VERY MUCH | AGREE SLIGHTLY | NEUTRAL | DISAGREE SLIGHTLY | DISAGREE VERY MUCH | TOTALLY DISAGREE |
|---|---|---|---|---|---|---|

22. I have to make sure other people are protected from all of the consequences of things I do.

| TOTALLY AGREE | AGREE VERY MUCH | AGREE SLIGHTLY | NEUTRAL | DISAGREE SLIGHTLY | DISAGREE VERY MUCH | TOTALLY DISAGREE |
|---|---|---|---|---|---|---|

23. Other people should not rely on my judgement.

| TOTALLY AGREE | AGREE VERY MUCH | AGREE SLIGHTLY | NEUTRAL | DISAGREE SLIGHTLY | DISAGREE VERY MUCH | TOTALLY DISAGREE |
|---|---|---|---|---|---|---|

24. If I cannot be certain I am blameless, I feel that I am to blame.

| TOTALLY AGREE | AGREE VERY MUCH | AGREE SLIGHTLY | NEUTRAL | DISAGREE SLIGHTLY | DISAGREE VERY MUCH | TOTALLY DISAGREE |
|---|---|---|---|---|---|---|

25. If I take sufficient care then I can prevent any harmful accidents.

| TOTALLY AGREE | AGREE VERY MUCH | AGREE SLIGHTLY | NEUTRAL | DISAGREE SLIGHTLY | DISAGREE VERY MUCH | TOTALLY DISAGREE |
|---|---|---|---|---|---|---|

26. I often think that bad things will happen if I am not careful enough.

| TOTALLY AGREE | AGREE VERY MUCH | AGREE SLIGHTLY | NEUTRAL | DISAGREE SLIGHTLY | DISAGREE VERY MUCH | TOTALLY DISAGREE |
|---|---|---|---|---|---|---|

Salkovskis P.M., Wroe A.L., Gledhill A., Morrison N., Forrester E., Richards C., Reynolds M. & Thorpe S. (2000), 'Responsibility attitudes and interpretations are characteristic of obsessive compulsive disorder', *Behaviour Research and Therapy*, 38, 347–372.

## OTHER PSYCHOLOGICAL VULNERABILITIES

Research has shown that ideas about responsibility are particularly important in the understanding of how OCD takes and keeps hold. However, other factors have been highlighted as playing a role for some people in their OCD.

## PERFECTIONISM

Most people want to achieve what they can in life and there are a range of ways that we go about motivating ourselves to do better – two important aspects of our progress through life are choosing and setting the right goals and how we feel when we meet, or sometimes fail to meet, those goals. Most people drive themselves very hard to do 'perfectly' some things they regard as 'important', and therefore set very high standards in the belief that this will help them achieve the best. This is generally fine, when the high standards are like ambitions, something the person is happy if they achieve and not too much of a problem if they don't. However, some people have perfectionistic standards for everything – not just the important piece of work that they are doing, but small things like how they carry out their everyday routines. What can then make it worse is if the perfectionistic standards are not a source of satisfaction, but instead a constant source of fear. Another problem with perfectionism is a type of 'putting all your eggs in one basket'. That is, the person who believes that everything depends on getting things right in one area of their life (and therefore much of their behaviour is motivated by the fear of getting things wrong in that area).

Positive perfectionism is when we persist in things which are important to us, allowing ourselves to apply lower standards in other areas. We can enjoy the rewards of a good job done well, and easily tolerate the imperfect trivia. However, if we treat everything as equally important and try to do everything perfectly, we are doomed to a negatively motivated perfectionistic life of slavery linked to our blindly high standards, and may be tortured by our fears of things going wrong (meaning, things which are not perfect). In OCD, not getting things we believe we have a responsibility for 'just right' turns out to be at the centre of things.

When people don't manage to meet the standards they set themselves, this might be a reason to try ever harder. Sometimes, however, the better response is to lower your standards so that they are achievable, and to choose carefully where we need to put our efforts. In summary, people who are vulnerable to experiencing a lot of psychological distress have particularly high standards about what they feel they should achieve and are motivated by fear of not meeting those standards rather than satisfaction if they do.

## VIEWS OF OURSELVES AND SELF-CRITICISM

Important factors that can either protect us against difficulties, or may make us more vulnerable to them, is how we view ourselves and our ability to look after ourselves mentally when we encounter difficulties. Many of us can tend to be self-critical with the underlying view that this will help us get where we want to be and that not to be self-critical will somehow make us fail in our efforts. This self-critical message usually has its origins in childhood or early experiences and has been reinforced over time by being harsh towards yourself. However, over time the effect of this may be to make us feel less capable and may undermine our self-confidence in important ways. When you hear the crowd at a football match they will usually shout out supportive things for their own team. However, if a member of the opposing team comes near they will shout out lots of negative things. The purpose of this is to undermine that player's confidence and make them play less well. So, if you are constantly criticising yourself and telling yourself that you are terrible, bad or stupid for making a mistake or doing compulsions, the overall effect of this will be that you will feel worse about yourself. This is likely to make the OCD seem more powerful. On the other side of the coin, if you take a more understanding and supportive approach to your problems, it may be that this will help you make more progress.

## BELIEFS ABOUT THE IMPORTANCE OF THOUGHTS

As with other types of beliefs, those about the importance of thoughts are there, even if we have never spent any time considering them. If we believed that 'thoughts don't mean anything at all' we would be less likely to be seriously troubled by a random intrusive thought. As we have discussed, people with OCD are very 'tuned in' to their thoughts and tend to make certain interpretations or assumptions about their thoughts, even if these are not articulated:

- That negative intrusive thoughts indicate something significant about yourself (that you are bad, weird, dangerous)
- That having the thoughts increases the risk of bad things happening (see 'Superstition and magical thinking' on page 61)
- That negative intrusive thoughts must be important merely because they have occurred

The esteemed psychologist Professor Stanley Jack Rachman, an expert in this area, gives some examples of attaching undue importance to the occurrence of intrusive thoughts:

- This thought reflects my true evil nature
- Having this thought means I'm a bad person
- If I think this, I must really want it to happen
- Thinking this can make the event more likely to happen
- If others knew I thought this, they would think I was an evil person
- Having this thought means I am likely to lose control over my mind or my behaviour

It follows that if you have beliefs such as these about your thoughts, you will want to try to do something to have fewer of the thoughts in the first place, and will also try to do something about them once they have occurred.

# TRIGGERING EVENTS AND CRITICAL INCIDENTS

If people have a number of underlying psychological and biological vulnerability factors, then for particular individuals an obsessional problem may start to develop when they encounter situations in life which bring these factors to the fore. In particular, situations which increase a person's sense of responsibility, or decrease their sense of control over their environment, are often significant in bringing ideas of responsibility to the fore. This can happen gradually, for example gaining more and more responsibility in work, or the ongoing effect of being bullied at school, but it can also happen quite suddenly, for example leaving home or becoming a parent for the first time. Good things can make us more worried; we may begin to notice that we have a lot more to lose than we previously realised. As discussed in Chapter 1, the key factor is how the person responds to these events, and how the events interact with their underlying beliefs and general assumptions about themselves, how the world works in general and their possible futures.

For example, the birth of a child may lead to OCD in someone who believes that they should take every possible precaution to ensure that they do not cause, or risk, harm to those who cannot protect themselves. They may not previously have been exposed to such high levels of (very real) responsibility. Suddenly, when they ask themselves 'What's the worst thing that could happen?', the answer seems very frightening.

Given the idiosyncratic nature of OCD, the particular triggering event, or events, can also be very individual. Common triggering events are changing school, other major life transitions like leaving home, losing a loved one, illness in yourself or someone important to you, having a baby, parental conflict, bullying, and relationship break-up. These events would, of course, be stressful for anyone, but for people who go on to develop OCD, there are often particular conclusions drawn at the time in relation to responsibility and the need to control what is happening. Sometimes there is no obvious triggering event, but a person experiences a worrying thought that they had never experienced or noticed before, and feels compelled to act. In either case, underlying responsibility beliefs play a role.

## CONTAMINATION ... AND MORE

The development of contamination fears has always seemed easy to understand; after all, we are bombarded by ideas of how best to wash our hands, avoid infection and other health and safety messages. However, there is a further type of contamination fear which is much harder to understand: this is called 'mental contamination'. In mental contamination, the person does not believe themselves to have picked up germs or poison, but feels inwardly polluted; dirty on the inside. Recently, one of the most important psychologists in the field, Professor Jack Rachman, pointed out the link between feelings of mental contamination and important formative experiences, particularly the experience of abuse and trauma from trusted people. He suggested that the experience of betrayal, a violation of trust by some person or organisation that we thought we could depend upon, can lead to feelings of mental contamination. It seems that we can feel contaminated and dirty because we have been *treated like dirt* when we were trusting. This feeling is dealt with by attempts to wash away the feeling; of course, because the feeling is inside, the washing fails.

## COURSE OF OCD

OCD can creep in over a number of years or can develop quite suddenly. Sometimes it can get better if circumstances change, but can recur at a later point. There are many reasons why people may not seek help straight away but one of them is that the obsessions and compulsions may seem at first to be helpful. Who can argue that taking care and being responsible is not a good thing? Of course it is not the taking care that is the problem, it is the fact that it becomes out of proportion to the risks involved. This is particularly tricky if you begin to view yourself as a potential risk to others. As we said before, the driving mechanisms of OCD are understandable as extreme versions of normal psychological processes. It may take a while for the behaviours to become extreme and obviously unhelpful, and sometimes it can be hard to identify exactly where this line is (and of course there is no real line). It may take a while, too, to realise that what you are doing has become very out of step with the norm, particularly if you are very focused on your own behaviour. It is not uncommon for others who know the person well to notice this well ahead of the person themselves. It makes sense that if you feel that your compulsions or avoidance are keeping you and others safe, it may feel like you have no choice but to continue doing them, or that it is a price worth paying.

In some cases, the symptoms which later turn into OCD may even start off as comforting, a kind of false friend. Little rituals can be soothing when they remain within limits. For some people, washing or checking or putting things in particular order makes them feel more in control at first. Only when these rituals take over and dominate do things begin to become problematic; as we describe below, 'the solution becomes the problem'.

Another aspect that can keep people suffering for a long time is not knowing what OCD is and how it works. If you have never heard of this problem or the fact that negative thoughts are normal and suddenly notice an intrusive thought or have an image of stabbing someone for example, it is very understandable that you might conclude that it means something terrible about you. Perhaps you may think that you may actually do it or that having the thought means you are going crazy. As well as causing a lot of anxiety, these types of interpretations may make you hesitant to seek help, and often it is the case that people struggle with such

## HOW DID MY PROBLEM DEVELOP?

It is natural to want to understand how your problem developed. However, due to the fact that the problem may have been influenced by things you experienced long ago – before you could even make sense of them – and that there are many factors which can have an influence on OCD, it is important to bear in mind that there may be no definite answers. However, it can be helpful to think of things that might be relevant, as this will help you identify and understand particular ideas and behaviours that keep your problem going in the present. Think back to when symptoms of the problem began to emerge (it may have been long after this that you began to consider that they were actually part of a problem).

Was there anything when you were growing up that made you more prone to being concerned about bad things happening?

Think about experiences, or patterns of experiences, where you may have had too much responsibility or were given too little. You may have been overprotected by parents or perhaps had to care for them in certain ways. Perhaps you had a time where you felt that things were very out of control, for example being bullied, or your parents breaking up.

Did anything happen that made you particularly concerned about taking risks or worry more about bad things happening?

Did you have any experiences that seemed to mean that you were capable of causing or preventing harm?

What ideas do you think you absorbed about harm and your role to prevent it?

What ideas did you internalise about what sort of person you are?

thoughts for a long time before finding out that these experiences are part of OCD. Shame and stigma can prevent you disclosing thoughts or symptoms even to your closest friends and family.

## SUMMARY

There is no one reason or set of reasons for developing OCD and we are each unique in our personality, our biological make-up and the set of experiences we have had. Therefore it is usually very hard to pinpoint the exact reasons why any one person develops a problem. Luckily it is not essential to know this in order to beat the problem, although it does no harm to spend a little time thinking about how we got to where we are with a problem like this. Nevertheless, it is much more important to focus on the 'here and now' and what is keeping the problem going at the moment. Although we may not know exactly what 'caused them', we know that currently held beliefs about responsibility and about the world in general help us understand why people find it hard to ignore, or dismiss, negative thoughts. The next chapter will help you understand how OCD takes hold and keeps hold.

# 3
# HOW DOES OCD TAKE HOLD AND KEEP HOLD?

The previous chapter outlined how the problem of OCD might develop given particular background factors and particular experiences. This chapter will build on this understanding by bringing the focus back into the here and now to help you think about:

- Exactly how you are stuck in a problem that is causing you distress
- What are the particular things you are doing, feeling and believing that are keeping the problem going

Realising that you have a problem is certainly the first step in doing something about it; however, it is not the only step. People with obsessional worries and compulsive behaviours are often told to 'just stop doing it' or to 'pull themselves together'. Oh, if only it were so easy. We have never ever met anyone with OCD who did not want, with all their heart, to just stop doing it. The problem for them is simple: how can they do so? We believe that, once someone knows in detail what they need to do, and have the right kind of support in place to help them do it, then they can and will 'pull themselves together'. Indeed, that is pretty much the only way to deal with OCD; getting rid of it, with or without professional and other input, has to be something which is done by the sufferer, through blood, toil, tears and sweat.

When people tell the OCD suffer to 'stop it', this does not take into account the reason why the drive to carry out obsessional behaviours is so strong – the deep and crucially important under-lying meaning that your intrusive thoughts have for you. If it were easy to stop acting on your fears, then clearly you would have done so already. However, there may have been times where you consid-ered your obsessional behaviour in the cold light of day and thought that 'I know it seems ridiculous but I really feel like I *have* to wash/check/do a ritual to keep safe'. So why is it that you are continuing to do things that at other times feel unreasonable?

The key part here is the idea that 'at other times' the behaviour seems unreasonable or the worry seems unfeasible. It is important to ask yourself, when you are *actually* washing/checking or doing any of your 'compulsive' behaviours, does it feel 'ridiculous' then? If you are stuck in a pattern of obsessional thoughts and behaviours, the answer is invariably 'no'. Generally, the compulsions *feel* neces-sary; doing them feels like a small price to pay to avert something bad happening and also offers the added benefit of giving you some relief from the mounting anxiety. The next part of the puzzle is to look at what is going on in detail when you are under the power of OCD and think about how and why the problem keeps going.

## RESPONSIBILITY APPRAISALS/BELIEFS ABOUT YOUR THOUGHTS

In Chapter 1, we learned that intrusive thoughts are normal and very common. So if lots of people are having the same types of thoughts, why is it so hard for you just to ignore or dismiss these thoughts? This is one of the most important ideas to understand when tackling your OCD. The difference between someone who is bothered by a thought and someone who is not lies in *what they make* of having the thought. For the first person, *having the thought itself* is interpreted as being particularly significant and it is this which causes both anxiety (an emotional response) and the need to do something about it (behavioural response – a compul-sion or avoidance).

> **KEY IDEA**
> It is the personal meaning of the thoughts that makes them so unpleasant, anxiety-provoking and difficult to dismiss. It's not the thoughts that are the problem; it's what you make of them.

If you have thoughts of violence or harm it may feel difficult to believe that the thoughts themselves are not intrinsically bad – you just don't want to have these thoughts and their very presence in your mind makes you anxious, upset, maybe disgusted or depressed. However, it is crucial to remember that anyone and everyone can have these kinds of thoughts. For example, it is *very unusual* for new mothers and fathers *not* to have thoughts of harming their baby, or of harm coming to it. The most upsetting intrusive thoughts are about our worst fears. This is, of course, also true of other types of thoughts such as those about contamination and safety; really, we are worrying about dangers which might materialise. In these cases it is still true that it is what you make of having the thought that makes it very difficult to ignore.

Think again of when you felt very anxious and you had the intrusive thought. Ask yourself all or some of the following questions:

- What is the worst thing that could happen?
- And, if that were to be true, what, for you, is particularly bad about that? (Every time you get an answer to that question, ask it again until you keep getting the same answer – see the example below)
- What is the worst thing about having this thought at all?
- What does this mean about me as a person that I have these thoughts at all?

Let's consider an example:

Intrusive thought: 'Have I left the front door open?'

*Question: What's the worst thing that could happen?*
Answer: 'Someone could break in.'
*Question: If that happens, what's so bad about that?*
Answer: 'Someone could steal my identity.'
*Question: What's so bad about that?*
Answer: 'They will commit a terrible crime of which I will be accused.'
*Question: What's the worst thing about that?*
Answer: 'I will not be able to prove that it was not me.'
*Question: What's the worst thing about that?*
Answer: 'I will go to prison, where I will be gang-raped.'

When we keep asking questions such as 'What's the worst thing about that?' we find out a very serious frightening idea. If you think you are going to be gang-raped in prison, it makes sense to go back and check your front door to prevent that from happening.

The answer to these questions will help you access the personal meaning that the thoughts have for you. It may take a bit of thinking to identify the meaning of the thoughts. Many people just focus on the thoughts themselves and move quickly to do something about it rather than reflecting on the deepest meaning that the thoughts have. However, it is this meaning which leads to the responses, even if we are not completely aware of it at all times.

Let's think again about some examples of intrusive thoughts and in further detail at possible appraisals that could lead to significant anxiety. In the table below, we show not only the meaning but the compulsion motivated by the meaning.

| INTRUSIVE THOUGHT | APPRAISAL: What is the worst thing about having this thought? What is the worst thing that could happen? What does this mean about me as a person to have these thoughts? | COMPULSIONS |
|---|---|---|
| **Thought** | | |
| 'There might be blood in my food' | I could catch a disease and die. This is the most frightening thing that I can imagine – I will die painfully, slowly and everyone will reject me. I must make sure that there is no chance of coming into contact with blood or other bodily fluids | Check all food carefully for anything unusual or ambiguous. Ensure that packaging has not been interfered with. Avoid anything where I have any doubt about its origin |
| 'That is contaminated with germs' | I might be responsible for spreading contamination. I will pass the disease to the children. This is the worst thing I could do as a parent. I need to make sure that this doesn't happen or I will never forgive myself, nor will anyone else | Wash self and home. Make sure that no 'dirty' objects come into contact with objects that are 'clean'. Avoid going anywhere where I can't keep track of what is clean and dirty. Wear gloves. Use alcohol gel whenever out |
| 'My appointment is on Friday 13th' | Something bad might happen if I go. This bad luck could last for a lifetime | Change the appointment. Wear 'lucky trousers' to the rearranged appointment |
| 'Did I run someone over without realising it?' | I could be a killer – reckless drivers are the worst of the worst – I cannot afford to take the risk | Go back and check. Listen out for unusual noises when driving. Avoid driving whenever possible |

| INTRUSIVE THOUGHT | APPRAISAL | COMPULSIONS |
|---|---|---|
| 'Have I left the front door open?' | Someone could break in and steal everything and it would be my fault. Someone will steal my identity, commit a terrible crime of which I will be accused. I will not be able to prove that it was not me – I will go to prison where I will be gang-raped. I must make sure there is no chance that anyone can break in | Go back and check. Install six locks. Spend half an hour each time making sure they are all locked. Take photo of the locked door. Pick up all my post directly from the post office to make sure no one is stealing it |

**Images**

| | | |
|---|---|---|
| Mum dead in a car crash | This could be a premonition. Thinking this means it will happen. Only a bad person would have these thoughts. I need to think something good – if I don't a bad thing will happen and it will all be my fault | Cross fingers and think of a positive image of her happy and well. Pray that nothing bad happens. Do what I did last time – count to 636 in multiples of six to make sure that nothing bad happens |
| Abusing a baby or child | Having this thought must mean that I am a monster. I need to make sure there is no risk that I can ever harm a child; if I ever did touch a child I would have to kill myself | Avoid all children, including walking past schools or children's shops. Make sure that I am not turned on when around children by checking for signs of arousal. Ask for reassurance that I haven't been anywhere on my own. Think back to times when I have been with children and try to remember whether anything inappropriate happened |

| INTRUSIVE THOUGHT | APPRAISAL | COMPULSIONS |
|---|---|---|
| **Urges** | | |
| 'I must touch that or I won't feel right' | I could feel uncomfortable for ever. I would not be able to cope with this; I must make sure that this doesn't happen or I will end up in a psychiatric hospital for the rest of my life | Touch it in groups of seven until feeling goes. Look up symptoms of severe mental illness on the internet |
| To jump in front of a train | I might be crazy – only someone mad would think such a thing | Never sit near platform edge. Avoid using train – use four buses instead. Monitor other thoughts for signs of madness |
| To physically assault someone | I am capable of doing something terrible – I shouldn't take the risk, I must protect myself and other people | Sit on hands. Read newspaper articles on recent murderers and abusers and check for similarities between them and me. Never go out alone. Go over the evidence in my head about whether I am a good or a bad person |

In all these examples, having the thought means something terrible. This is unpleasant enough; however, OCD doesn't stop there. You will note in all the examples above a fundamental process in OCD that we discussed in Chapter 2: *taking responsibility* for preventing anything bad happening – 'I must make sure that nothing bad happens' – which drives all the compulsions (safety-seeking behaviours or neutralising).

**KEY IDEA**

People with OCD think and feel an acute sense of responsibility to:

- Prevent harm
- Prevent something bad happening to themselves or others
- Make amends if they think something bad might have already happened as a result of their thoughts or actions

This idea of responsibility is the link or bridge between the intrusive thoughts and the responses to them, particularly the ritualising and neutralising.

The sense of responsibility fuels anxiety – who wouldn't be anxious if they thought something bad was happening and they could do something to stop it? It makes a great deal of sense that once this responsibility belief is around, people with OCD feel a great need to perform compulsions, rituals or safety-seeking behaviours. We will go on to consider the counterproductive nature of these attempts to reduce the thoughts and discharge the responsibility. Responsibility appraisals can distort your perceptions of how likely, important or awful something is.

## PROBABILITY AND 'AWFULNESS'

An important idea that keeps OCD going is that even if something bad happening is unlikely, you should still do everything possible to try to prevent it (i.e. inflated responsibility belief). So the probability or likelihood of something bad happening interacts with how awful it would be if it did happen. That is to say, it might not happen but if it did it would be *so* terrible that my life would effectively be over, *and* I could have prevented it! For example, the person who feels contaminated worries that their hands have HIV on them. It may not seem very likely, but if they really are contaminated, then there is some chance that their children will get infected, become ill and later die horribly, when all they needed to do was a little washing. Obviously, washing in these circumstances makes *short term* sense ... what's the problem with washing when the stakes seem so high?

There is nothing wrong or unusual with taking responsibility for preventing something bad happening. Most people would take steps to prevent accidents or harm coming to themselves or others. Examples could be installing locks on the front door, driving carefully, reporting a gas leak, not dropping banana skins on the street and not serving a friend rotten food. However, most people are able to make do with only one lock on the door, don't spend time every day checking for gas leaks or the presence of banana skins. This is because while most people think that 'bad things' *can* happen, they don't believe that they are particularly likely or probable, and if they did happen, they think that it might not be that bad, or that they would deal with it if it happened. That is, even if there was a gas leak, it is unlikely that anyone will die; even if someone did slip on a banana skin, they would get a bruise rather than a broken neck. People with OCD go to great lengths to avoid bad things happening. They tend to focus on the worst possible thing, focusing on how awful it would be if it did happen. People with OCD feel that what they fear *is* likely to happen and are very motivated to avoid the possibility that they could be responsible if they did not try to prevent it happening. The above situations are more examples of 'the solution becoming the problem'.

---

### KEY IDEA: THE TOXIC TRIO
People with OCD think that bad things:
- Are likely to happen
- Would be very awful if they did happen
- Are their responsibility to prevent happening

---

Think of the examples of appraisals on pages 56–58 – if you really thought that those bad things could happen, what would you do? Perhaps some of the examples are similar to your own concerns – what have you found yourself doing?

## SUPERSTITION AND MAGICAL THINKING

Some people with OCD describe what is sometimes called 'magical thinking' or, in one type of magical thinking, 'thought–action fusion'. This is driven by another common set of beliefs that can become more extreme in OCD. For example, many people believe that saying or thinking something bad about someone else makes it more likely that something bad will happen, for example 'tempting fate'. Most people are brought up to not say 'bad things' about others, often with a cultural or religious undercurrent that there will some negative consequences should they do so. Magical thinking in OCD is an extension of this very mainstream thinking – the belief that unpleasant, unacceptable thoughts can influence events in the world. Magical thinking in OCD is an extension of this very mainstream thinking – the belief that unpleasant, unacceptable thoughts can influence events in the world. It fits with things like superstitions, belief in horoscopes and so on.

Interestingly, despite the strong cultural message that saying or thinking certain words is 'unlucky' or might 'jinx' things, or that crossing your fingers means that something 'doesn't count', most people also accept that this couldn't possibly work for positive events. For example, buying a lottery ticket and saying 'I'm going to win tonight' doesn't make it more likely that the numbers will come up. In fact, most people also accept that this doesn't really work for negative events – if thinking about someone dying actually made them die, people with OCD would be in demand as assassins! Think how easy it would be to get rid of dictators or serial killers if we could just imagine them dying.

**RESEARCH NOTE**

Two world experts in OCD coined the phrase 'thought–action fusion' and identified two main themes in this thinking:

- **Likelihood thought-action fusion**: the belief that having an unwanted, unacceptable thought increases the likelihood that a specific adverse event will occur, i.e. if I think about falling ill, it makes it more likely that I will become ill

- **Moral thought-action fusion**: the belief that having an unacceptable intrusive thought is almost the moral equivalent of carrying out that particular act, i.e. if I think about swearing in church, this is almost as bad as actually swearing in church

Shafran, R. & Rachman, S. (2004), 'Thought-action fusion: a review', *Journal of Behavior Therapy and Experimental Psychiatry*, 35, 87-107.

## NOT TRUSTING YOUR SENSES/DOING SOMETHING UNTIL IT 'FEELS RIGHT'

Consider locking the front door. Most people turn the key, the lock makes a clunking noise and they walk away without thinking anything more about it. However, it all seems a bit different if you suffer from OCD and this focuses on checking doors and the threats of not having properly locked up. Typically in this type of OCD, people stop trusting their senses, doubt their memory for what they have done and abandon their usual ways of deciding that they have performed an action. So when locking the front door, people with OCD might doubt whether they actually did turn the key and hear the clunk, wondering whether they were, instead, actually remembering locking the door yesterday. They may try to remember more clearly, or try to remember whether they saw the door wide open as they walked away. To try to be more certain, they may repeatedly push at the door before leaving, look back at the door while walking down the street, repeatedly saying today's date, taking a picture of the door on their camera phone in case of later doubt and, if that is not enough, to go back and check if they are still not certain. Other similar aspects of the problem are 'getting it just right' or doing something until it 'feels right'. This could include ordering the cupboards in a particular way, getting up and down from a chair, saying prayers or washing hands.

It almost seems like they are making these decisions as if their life depended on it. In fact, that is the key to understanding the desire to keep repeating obsessional actions until 'it feels just right'. Most people don't focus on how they feel about something and use that feeling to decide whether to make the decision to stop checking or washing their hands and other 'ordinary' decisions. However, people do use their feelings to decide whether they know enough, are sure enough or have done enough *for very important decisions*. Think about taking a new job, getting married, moving to a new house. How do you decide? Well, to make that kind of decision, most people gather all the information they can get, they go over it again and again; they get advice from other people, they test it out in any way they can and keep going *until it feels right*. If it *doesn't* feel right, then the person will decide that, contrary to the evidence, they should keep at it until they feel much more sure. Now most people don't do this for things like stopping washing their hands or checking the door or mentally checking things out for the simple reason that most people don't think that these things are a matter of life or death. However, people with OCD do, and as a result, treat decisions like when to stop washing and checking like other people do for very very important decisions. As described above, for the person with OCD deciding when to stop *is* a very very important decision, so they put all their efforts into the attempt to be completely sure before they can move on to the next thing they need to do. So, it's not surprising that people with OCD take so long to complete things connected to their obsessional fears. The person with contamination fears is, from their point of view, making a life-or-death decision when they decide that they are clean enough.

Research tells us, unfortunately, that these ways of making a decision (by repeating things over and over) has the odd effect of making us less confident about the thing that we are checking. This is probably because our memory becomes less clear as we repeat things; which occasion are we remembering? The first time or the 20th time? However, if we do things once only, then our memory will typically be clearer. We remember reasonably confidently when we do things once; when we repeat things, our confidence gets progressively lower. Notice that the research tells us that this is true for everyone, and the people with OCD are not different from those without, *except* that people with OCD are much much more likely than everyone else to repeat things in this way.

An added problem is that, having tried once to be completely certain, this tends to make us feel that it is sufficiently important to try to do the same thing again and again and again. Having found it difficult before, it is no surprise that it is difficult the next time. For example, if you check the door for half an hour on Monday, you can't get away with checking it for ten minutes on Tuesday – usually only the full half-hour will feel right, and usually more and more time is required to get the 'just right' feeling. As OCD continues, the person finds that they get less satisfaction about whether things are right or not for more and more time, but for practical reasons they have to finish before things feel right, making them feel more and more uneasy. This is yet another of the pernicious vicious circles which are involved in turning normal worries into crippling OCD.

## IMPOSSIBLE CRITERIA AND THE NEED FOR CERTAINTY

We sometimes refer to 'impossible criteria' in OCD. This is when the problem asks you to do something that is actually impossible

– i.e. to be sure that something is 100% clean, to be 100% certain. As this is unachievable, no amount of checking, washing or repeating will ever be enough. Furthermore, trying to be completely certain of something makes you look for any 'chinks in the armour' of certainty. Given that certainty is a feeling, this process is bound to increase doubt.

We all feel more stable in conditions of certainty. It helps to know that we have enough money coming in, that we can trust that our loved ones are generally there for us, that we have a roof over our heads and are generally well. However, if we said that we had to be completely, 100% certain of those things before we could do anything, we would no doubt struggle greatly. We live life according to our best assumptions and deal with problems when they occur.

One of the most difficult versions of this problem involves checking our memory. Most people with OCD are particularly worried about whether or not they have done something to harm others; for example, you may be concerned that you might have knocked someone over when you walked or drove past. To make sure that you have *not* done so, you look back the way you came … was someone lying on the ground? Later, you go over this memory in your mind again and again … are you really sure that there was no one injured? Do you have a clear memory that there was nothing going on behind you? How clear is your recollection? The problem here is that we can never have a clear recollection of something that didn't happen or that we didn't see … how could we? But, if you suffer from OCD, you really want to be completely clear and certain.

If you don't have a clear memory, how certain can you possibly be? As you try again and again to form a clear memory of what didn't happen, as with other types of memory, repeated checking of the memory makes you less and less confident about it. Linked to this is the attempt to reconstruct memory. There were 20 people standing in a group as you drove past … when you looked in your car mirror to try to make sure that you didn't hit any of them, you saw the group again. Later you try to remember ... all of them. Were they all there? What did they look like afterwards? Again, you are trying the impossible memory feat, and you are not only bound to fail, but also bound to be upset about not being sure. The more upset you get, the harder you try to be sure, the more confused you feel. Again, a range of vicious circles click in. None of these things is abnormal. Research on eyewitnesses shows that people have particular difficulties in recalling things which didn't happen. Unscrupulous lawyers know that if you question people ('were you 100% sure that he wasn't there?') doubts creep in, and the harder that a person is pushed about how sure they are, the more they begin to doubt. For the person with OCD, OCD is that unscrupulous lawyer, and to make it worse, it knows your innermost thoughts!

Notice that all of these problematic reactions are motivated not just by the fear of harm but by the fear of being responsible for harm, which in turn motivates enormous effort directed towards making sure that the person cannot be blamed for the feared disasters.

## AVOIDANCE

Avoidance is one of the most common strategies to deal with fears and to deal with growing obsessions and compulsions. At its worst, avoidance can utterly destroy a person's life, for example leading them to completely avoid their loved ones. OCD can make people become housebound, like being an agoraphobic, and avoidance can mean that the sufferer is completely paralysed, stuck in one position for literally hours on end. Equally, the avoidance can become both subtle and complicated, so that although it consumes the person's entire time and effort, the outside observer would notice little wrong.

## THE COUNTERPRODUCTIVE NATURE OF COMPULSIONS/RITUALS/ NEUTRALISING OR SAFETY-SEEKING BEHAVIOURS AND AVOIDANCE

In the table on pages 56–58 we can see how it makes sense to engage in all sorts of physical and mental actions or avoidance to feel safe, better or less anxious, or to 'neutralise' (cancel something out) as a result of the sense of responsibility, and to try to get rid of the thoughts themselves. All washing, checking, counting, praying, asking for reassurance, avoiding, have come about in the first place to try to make you feel safer and less anxious, but in fact do the exact opposite. Even if they provide temporary relief from anxiety, all these physical and mental behaviours **make the meaning attached to those intrusive thoughts, images, urges and doubts feel more true**, and therefore keep the need to do the behaviours going, making the meaning feel even more true and so on.

---

**KEY IDEA**

There are some big problems with compulsions:

- By responding to the belief that you are responsible, you implicitly accept the implication of being responsible in the first place
- Compulsions focus you on the responsibility belief and the intrusive thoughts themselves, making the thoughts more accessible and noticeable in your thinking
- You become more anxious and preoccupied
- **You do not get the chance to find out what would happen if you didn't do the compulsions**

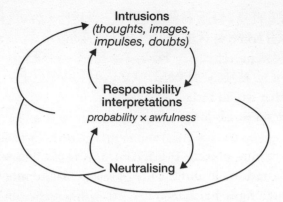

Think of the last time that you were engaged in some kind of physical or mental compulsion, and ask yourself the following questions:

- At that time, what was the effect of reacting that way on your belief that something bad could happen (and that it was your responsibility to do something about it)?
- As you felt anxious, did you believe this more or less, and did your compulsions feel more or less important?
- Has it ever permanently got rid of an obsessional worry?
- Have you ever thought that all this stuff you do might be making the problem worse?

---

**KEY IDEA**

'The solution becomes the problem' – the more you buy in to the idea that you are responsible, the compulsions become more important/time consuming/repetitive.

---

Let's look at some common compulsions and examine how all these things keep the problem going and make it worse.

## RITUALS

Rituals can come in many guises – there is no limit to their variety and complexity. They may be related to the fear in a very obvious way, or may develop a very individual connection with the fear that would be hard for others to guess.

Common rituals include:

- Touching objects in a certain way a specified number of times or in multiples of a particular number, e.g. touching a light switch seven times or seven times seven times
- Avoiding certain colours or deliberately wearing certain colours, e.g. not wearing black due to a belief that it is associated with evil
- Routine or ordering – having to get dressed in a particular set order; starting again if you make a mistake
- Cancelling out bad thoughts with good thoughts

The problem with rituals is that:

- ➤ Engaging in them 'buys in' to the idea that you are responsible for preventing something bad happening
- ➤ They only provide a temporary relief from anxiety
- ➤ They become more elaborate and lengthy over time

If you don't do your rituals, you find out what would actually happen – whether your fears would come true.

## CHECKING

Checking is a very common manifestation of OCD. Some of the many things that people check include:

- That the front door is locked
- That the baby is breathing
- That appliances are switched off

- That they haven't committed a terrible crime – checking newspapers or the internet for reports of a crime; calling the police to ask if anyone has been attacked or murdered
- Checking for signs of sexual arousal when around children
- That no one in the family has had an accident

Think about the things that you check – have you had to check more or less as time has passed? The problem with checking is that:

➤ Over time, it is likely that you have had to check more, and in a more elaborate way
➤ By checking in the first place, you are treating your belief about responsibility as true, making it feel more true with each check
➤ As you continue checking, in order for it to 'feel' right or be 'enough' and for you to stop feeling anxious you end up doing more and more
➤ It becomes harder to stop, as each time you do your checking you 'buy in' to the idea that the checking was necessary to stop something bad happening

If you don't check, you find out what would actually happen – whether your fears would come true.

## Mental checking/mental argument/doubting

Mental checking works in a similar way to physical checking – repeated attempts to ensure that something has or hasn't happened. As we described in the 'not trusting your senses' section on page 62, conscious and deliberate efforts to mentally check in an effort to feel extra sure or remember exactly do not yield certainty – in fact this checking generates further doubt.

**IS THAT YOUR FINAL ANSWER?**

On *Who Wants To Be A Millionaire?*, when presenter Chris Tarrant says 'Are you sure? Is that your final answer?' – does that make the contestant feel less anxious? Or does that questioning make them feel less sure, and more anxious? Often contestants get more anxious and 'phone a friend' or display further doubt in their answer. OCD often makes people mentally check, or argue, with themselves, which has the effect of making them more uncertain.

Mental checking can sometimes involve trying to remember something that *didn't* happen – this is an example of an 'impossible criterion': trying to remember something that didn't happen is unachievable. The effort to try to do this generates further doubt and anxiety while making it feel more important to be certain. See 'Impossible criteria and the need for certainty' on page 64.

So there are some big problems with mental checking:

➤ It 'buys into' and strengthens the idea that you are responsible
➤ It provides only temporary relief from anxiety
➤ It stops you from finding out what would happen if you did not mentally check – that your anxiety would decrease
➤ It increases your sense of doubt
➤ It is effortful, often requiring more effort over time
➤ It increases emphasis on internally referenced subjective criteria – 'remembering clearly', 'feeling sure', 'getting it just right'

If you don't check, you find out what would actually happen – whether your fears would come true.

## Avoidance

OCD often tells people to avoid all sorts of things:

- Public toilets
- Children's playgrounds
- People with diseases
- Unlucky colours

---

**TRYING TO AVOID OR SUPPRESS THOUGHTS**

Trying to avoid thoughts themselves is a particularly powerful part of OCD. We illustrate this with the 'white polar bears' example:

Try as hard as you can not to think about white polar bears. Do **not** imagine their fluffy white faces, definitely **do not think** about their little cubs sliding about on the ice. **Don't** think about them.

What do you notice? For most people, it is extremely difficult to **not** think about something. You have to have an idea of something in order to push it out of your mind, which means that you are already thinking of it. In fact, generally trying to suppress a thought has the paradoxical effect of making it more noticeable.

So trying to avoid thoughts is not only difficult, but also usually futile and counterproductive.

---

Additionally, it is common to try to avoid triggers for intrusive thoughts.

The problem with avoidance is:

➤ It buys into and strengthens the idea that you are responsible

➤ You never have the chance to find out what really happens

➤ This makes the avoidance seem more important and difficult to change

➤ The list of things to avoid can get longer

If you don't avoid, you find out what would actually happen – whether your fears would come true.

## REASSURANCE

If you believe that you are responsible for harm, or capable of being a paedophile, or that you can't be trusted to lock your house, it seems like a good idea to ask someone if you have done anything too risky, whether you have sexually abused anyone while you were drunk, whether the door is locked, whether you are completely clean ... and so on. Reassurance is, again, something we all normally seek.

As children, we are constantly seeking and being given reassurance by those around us (teachers, parents and so on). It's helpful in building our confidence. Gradually we make the transition from seeking reassurance (where someone else takes responsibility for our concerns and tells us that all will be well) to seeking support, where we have taken our own decisions (and have responsibility for them) but the other person provides emotional support, showing confidence in us and acceptance that, even if things go wrong, they will stand by us. However, even as adults, when things are anxiety-provoking, it is very good from our point of view to have someone else step in and share the responsibility for really difficult and threatening situations, whether that is our boss or a friend. So most people not only seek support but also, from time to time, reassurance when something seems especially threatening.

For the OCD sufferer, things which are easily manageable for others can seem particularly difficult and threatening, so they turn to the more confident for reassurance about whether their hands are clean, the door is locked, their thoughts are dangerous and so on. The fact that others appear confident about these things makes it easier to ask, and also easier for the other person to provide the reassurance. However, it is in the nature of OCD that the more reassurance you seek and get, the more you need. Bear in mind that reassurance seeking is a type of compulsive behaviour, simply a type of checking with others which has the added advantage of sharing responsibility with that other person. Checking as a way of dealing with obsessional fears can be compared to 'digging to get out of a hole'. Reassurance is similar, except that it's a bit like asking a trusted person to get down into the hole and dig alongside you as a way of trying to escape the hole.

So, there are a range of problems linked to asking for reassurance. The main effects of seeking reassurance are that:

➤ It buys into and strengthens the idea that you are responsible
➤ It only provides temporary relief from anxiety
➤ It stops you from finding out what would happen if you did not ask for reassurance – that your anxiety would decrease
➤ It makes you more inclined to seek reassurance the next time
➤ It increases your sense of doubt

Another significant drawback of reassurance is that it embroils others in your OCD. It is very difficult for family or friends to withhold reassurance if you are anxious or upset. However, it is often upsetting for others to become involved in this way – this might lead to arguments, breakdown of relationships and misery for all concerned. Unfortunately, they are helping your OCD rather than you when they give you reassurance. We know from research that at least in the *short term* the person seeking reassurance tends to feel better, and not asking for it (and not giving it) has the immediate effect of increasing anxiety. Typically, both the reassurance seeker and the person responding by giving feel that they have no other choice.

Ways of dealing with the urge to seek reassurance and, for the other person, responding to the reassurance seeking, will be discussed in Chapter 8.

If you don't ask for reassurance, you find out what would actually happen – whether your fears would come true.

## 'SELECTIVE ATTENTION' OR LOOKING FOR TROUBLE

OCD is an anxiety-related problem. One of the main effects of anxiety is to make the sufferer more sensitive to any sign of danger or threat. A good way of thinking about this is in terms of 'looking for trouble': if someone is anxious, then they scan everything they come across for signs of danger. This is actually helpful if you are in a dangerous situation (for example, walking in the jungle where there might be wild animals), because it prepares you to react really quickly once there is some sign that the danger might be about to strike. However, it is much less helpful when the

---

**'SELECTIVE ATTENTION' – ON THE LOOKOUT FOR TROUBLE:**

**Pigeons with bird AIDS**

Think of the last time you left the house and walked along the street. How many pigeons or other birds did you notice? A few? None?

Imagine now that you had just heard a radio broadcast that described a new and deadly form of a disease – bird AIDS. This can be transmitted to humans by contact with birds. How many birds are you likely to notice now? Most likely a lot more, as the birds now represent a risk or a threat to you. Your attention will be drawn to the birds.

This works in the same way for thoughts or 'triggers'. If you hold the belief that your thoughts are a sign of danger – that something bad is going to happen or that you are bad in some way – you will notice them more, and they will probably occur more.

---

danger is due to misinterpretation (thinking things are more dangerous than they really are). Unfortunately, OCD tunes you in to risk. It makes you more likely to spot 'risky' situations – and to notice those intrusive thoughts and things linked to them. This makes it seem as if the world really is a dangerous place; there are signs of possible danger everywhere, so anxiety increases, which further increases sensitivity to danger and so on. When you feel anxious and threatened, things which might or might not be signs of danger are pretty much always interpreted as indicating that danger really is just round the corner.

Selective attention works in the same way in the world around you. If you are 'tuned in' to dirt or germs, you will notice marks or stains on any- and everything that you touch.

Another thinking process that occurs in OCD is 'threat bias'. If you see something ambiguous, you are likely to assume that it is something bad rather than good. A useful example of this would be walking in long grass in a country that was populated by poisonous snakes. If you saw a long, thin, slightly coiled form on the ground, it would be quite likely that you would freeze on the spot or jump away as you jumped to the conclusion that it was a poisonous snake. In fact it could be another kind of snake, or a belt or rope that someone had dropped on the floor.

So in OCD, if you think that dirt or germs will kill you, as well as being more tuned in to noticing potential dirt or germs in the first place, you will make the assumption that ambiguous situations are dangerous. A small coffee stain looks brown, and if you are anxious about contamination, it can seem likely that it is blood. This links to general beliefs like 'It's better to be safe than sorry'. Someone who strongly holds such a belief will not take even the smallest risk. The trouble is, when you start to look for it, almost everything around us *could* be risky.

## SUMMARY

If you think you are responsible for preventing something bad happening, it makes sense to try to do something about it. People with OCD engage in a range of 'safety-seeking behaviours' including checking, reassurance seeking and avoiding. All these make the problem worse, by 'buying in to' the belief that you are responsible and prevent you finding out what would happen if you did not take these actions.

## THE 'VICIOUS FLOWER'

We have described above many of the main factors which contribute to turning normal intrusive thoughts experienced by everyone into the pattern of intrusions, their meaning and the way people react to this meaning which forms the trap which is OCD. We use a 'vicious flower' diagram to help us bring together the various ways of understanding what is involved in OCD.

The meaning attached to the thought, including that element of responsibility, forms the centre of the flower. This is because research tells us that this is the key meaning driving the problem.

An obvious impact of this responsibility belief is an increased focus on intrusive thoughts; the thoughts actually become more accessible in your mind, as do other related thoughts. For example, if you have a thought of something bad happening to your mum, you are also likely to think of something bad happening to your sister. Having thought about either or both and thought that they might mean that something terrible might happen because you thought these things, you become super sensitive to these thoughts coming again.

So we can draw out in a diagram the connection between ideas about harm and responsibility, the intrusive thought and the interpretation. As we get more intrusions, the appraisal may seem more likely, so we focus our attention on intrusions and so on. In this way, a vicious circle is set up, which is a key process in how OCD takes and keeps hold.

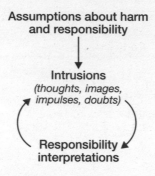

However, as we have explained, this is not the only vicious circle of reactions and behaviour which strengthen the central threatening meaning. The other vicious circles, or 'petals' are a way of showing how people with OCD react to that meaning, including not only how they feel but also what they do when that key meaning is activated. The responses include things that people do without thinking about it or making a choice (such as feeling anxious) as well as behaviours they engage in to prevent what they fear happening (such as rituals or avoidance). An arrow out connects the meaning with each of these responses. Perhaps most importantly, the arrows that go back into the centre completing each petal of the flower show that each of these is a vicious circle and so represent the counterproductive nature of safety-seeking behaviours. As well as reinforcing the responsibility belief, each process can also result in having more of the problematic intrusions.

If all of these things are going on at once, it's not surprising that you keep doing what you are doing. The vicious flower is a way of helping you understand how the complicated combination of vicious circles come together and interlock to fix OCD in place, resulting in the misery and disability which all too often takes over all parts of life. In Chapter 4 we will see how this framework applies to some particular case examples and how to use it to understand and beat your problem. By understanding and mapping out the processes that have been keeping the problem going we have a good guide to moving forward.

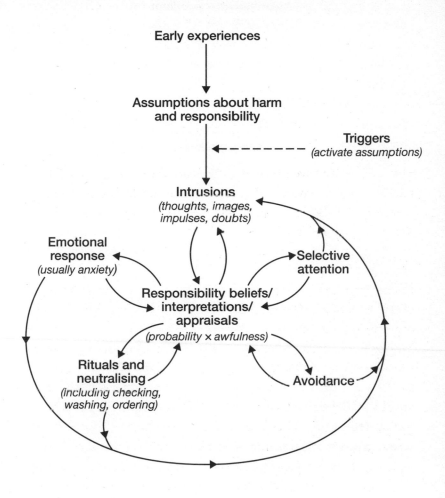

## TROUBLESHOOTING: THIS ISN'T HOW IT WORKS FOR ME ...

### 'I DON'T FEEL RESPONSIBLE FOR PREVENTING ANYTHING BAD HAPPENING'

You might be reading this thinking 'I don't feel responsible for preventing anything bad happening but I still spend hours every day checking/washing/ordering and avoiding many things'. It might be that you have had this problem for so long that you don't really know why you do the things you do. You might just feel that you 'have to' do certain things – but ask yourself what would be so bad when you do try to stop the rituals.

If it is still unclear, then try not doing the ritual and pay attention to what is going through your mind when you do so. Perhaps you have been doing them for so long that they have become detached from the meaning. But more likely, they are now such a habit that you have not thought about the meaning for some time. It could be that the meaning is quite frightening to really think about and that the rituals have served another purpose in stopping you thinking about things.

There is a lot of research about how this works with actions that we perform over and over again so that they become habitual. Psychologists call such behaviours 'proceduralised', which means that they are carried out with little or no effort by the person who has become used to doing them. We described an example of this in Chapter 1– the difference between a novice and experienced driver approaching traffic lights.

## My problem isn't about responsibility – it's about needing to be in control

Sometimes people describe 'needing to stay in control' rather than having beliefs about responsibility. The same question applies – what is so bad about not being in control? Why do you need to have control over your thoughts or control over what has touched what in your house? The same ideas apply – your need to have a feeling of control actually leads to you being out of control of your life, spending all your time doing washing/checking/ordering/counting.

## GOALS: GETTING BACK WHAT THE PROBLEM HAS BEEN TAKING FROM YOU, AND MORE

You might be reading this thinking 'but I really do need to keep going with my checking/washing/avoiding' as something bad really will happen, it would be truly awful and it would be my fault, therefore it is my responsibility to prevent it from happening'. This is common and it is not surprising to think this way, as OCD has a way of convincing you that all the things you do (or don't do) are a small price to pay. In Chapter 1 we asked you to think about the way this problem is affecting your life – how much time and money the problem costs you, the impact on your relationships and your ability to work and enjoy yourself. If OCD has affected any of these areas for you, something bad has already happened.

Considering the costs is a very important step in coming to terms with the fact that there is a problem to be tackled. But there is another reason for getting you to consider this: now is the time to think not only about how much the OCD has taken from you, but what should be the first targets for change to get your life back on track. Have another look at the list of areas where the problem has been affecting you:

- Time
- Money
- Ability to have emotional and physical intimacy
- Family members and friends
- Job/education

Think about all of these areas and what you would like to target in each. That is, if the OCD was to improve, what could you do again? Try to be as clear and concrete as possible. In this way, you will definitely know if you have achieved the goal. Thinking about what you want to be different in all aspects of your life is important to help you to stay focused on how you will break free from OCD. Think of what you would like to change straight away as well as things that will take a bit longer.

Of course it is completely reasonable to aim to 'feel better' but how would you know for sure if you had got there and made progress with the OCD? Would you be going out more with friends? Would you be able to take your children to the park to play in the sandpit? Would you be able to leave the house within 10 minutes? Would you be able to use a public loo?

Doing this will also remind you of the reasons that you are going through the anxiety of facing up to the OCD bully. Think what life will be like when you begin to claim it back.

# 4

# UNDERSTANDING YOUR PROBLEM

The last chapter described in detail the processes that OCD uses to take over. This chapter builds on your understanding by showing you how this works in particular forms of OCD. At the end of the chapter we will guide you through applying this to your own problem.

## CHECKING OCD

Checking is a normal part of life. We check things that we consider to be important, things that relate to avoiding particular negative consequences for ourselves or other people. The consequences might be in terms of physical danger (concern about accidents leading us to check a child's seatbelt), or social danger, that is, the way people view us (concern about judgement from our boss causing us to check our email asking for annual leave).

We are usually prompted to check by a thought, doubt or image occurring in our minds. For example, most people can recall a time when they were halfway down the street and they had a thought that they might have left the gas on, or the window open. They may even have gone back to check, especially if they were about to go off on holiday for two weeks. Then on the way to the airport, they suddenly have another intrusive thought ... did I remember my passport? So they check that too. In these circumstances checking can be helpful. It can make us feel happy that we can go secure in the knowledge that things are okay.

However if, even after we had checked the gas was safely off, we then went back to check again and again; something about the checking is no longer reassuring us. In OCD it is the *amount* and the *extent* of checking that determines whether or not there is a problem, not the fact that the person checks. Checking things repeatedly and painstakingly can quickly become a serious problem as it is usually very time-consuming and stressful.

There is no limit to the sort of things people might check obsessively, but most frequently the focus is on work, the home or accidentally having done something wrong. The content of the fears and checks can be very individual, depending on the situation the person is in.

| EXAMPLES OF THINGS PEOPLE CHECK | RELATED FEAR |
| --- | --- |
| Appliances, taps, stoves | This could catch fire |
| Locks, windows and doors | Someone could break in |
| Written work | I may make a mistake |
| Letters and emails | I may say something I didn't mean and embarrass myself |
| The road while driving | I may have knocked someone over without knowing it |
| Hospital drug charts | I may accidentally give a patient the wrong dose of medicine |

If you find that you are checking things over and over again on a daily basis, and this is interfering with your life then you may have the checking type of OCD.

**DO I HAVE CHECKING OCD?**
- Do you experience doubts, images or thoughts that things are unsafe?
- Do you check things repeatedly, even when you were sure they were fine the first time?
- Does the time spent checking make you late?
- Do you get anxious when you check?

## How does checking become a problem or 'better safe than sorry'?
### Background beliefs and trigger events

If it is normal to check, then how does checking become a problem? The particular ideas and beliefs we hold about ourselves and the world in general play a role in developing obsessional checking. Background beliefs such as 'deep down I am a careless person' are very common in people who have checking OCD. What follows from such a belief is that they may take extra care about things because they feel that they, even more than the average person, need to be particularly careful. This kind of belief may develop from past experiences such as having been in some way responsible for something going wrong, or feeling like you had a near miss. Subtle experiences such as being repeatedly told as a child that you are careless can lead to developing this sort of idea about yourself. In many cases we are not consciously aware of the beliefs we hold about certain issues as they may not be relevant in the particular circumstances we are in. Changes in life that entail more responsibility, like having a new home or job, can bring these beliefs to the fore. It is important to say here that you may not have experienced a specific event that triggered your OCD. For many people, the checking can increase gradually over a number of years until something or someone makes them question what they are doing.

### The meaning of thoughts: I can't ignore thoughts of danger

If you are someone who checks obsessively, it is likely that when you experience a doubt such as whether you turned something off, it will be very difficult for you to ignore or dismiss that concern. Sometimes the doubt can take the form of an image (of not having done it or of the things which might go wrong if you made a mistake). You may feel that you need to be completely certain that something is safe before you could get on with something else (see below). You might feel that it would be irresponsible to ignore such a thought as the consequences of doing so could be so terrible. The problem is that people with obsessive checking experience lots of these kind of doubts, even when they have just checked something. *Especially* when they have just checked something; as described above, we now know that checking can and does have the effect of undermining confidence in our memory.

### Better safe than sorry: the unassailable logic of checking

In a world where there are accidents and crime, it is reasonable to take care. People check, whether obsessively or not, in order to reduce the likelihood of certain bad things happening. However, if you are doing it repeatedly, then the checking is no longer fulfilling the function it was meant to.

If the checking was effective, then you would not need to check more than once. This is because performing repeated checks actually makes you feel *less* certain that you did something correctly. Experimental research studies show that asking anyone to check things repeatedly can cause them to experience more doubt about whether or not they had actually done it. So, if you begin to check things repeatedly and you also hold a belief that you must act on doubts in order to keep safe, a vicious circle of checking and doubting begins. This is the true paradox of checking repeatedly: checking actually makes people feel less certain and less safe.

A key part of the logic that keeps people checking is that the thing they fear *did not happen*, which they attribute to doing their checks. However, what doing the checks stops them from finding out is that this *would not have happened anyway.*

---

## ABSENCE OF EVIDENCE IS NOT EVIDENCE OF ABSENCE: THE MAN ON THE TRAIN

A man on the train to London stood by the window ripping up paper and throwing the pieces out of the window. A passenger asked him, *'Why are you doing that?'* Without stopping his task, he replied, *'It stops the elephants from stampeding on the track'.* The passenger replied, *'But there are no elephants on the track in London.'* *'Exactly!'* the man replied. *'It's working!'* And he carried on throwing the paper out of the window.

---

### Checking: impossible criteria

Think carefully about the last time you got stuck in a loop of repetitive checking: what was it that you were trying to achieve as you were doing the checks? Were you looking for a 'feeling' of certainty that things were safe? Often people wish to feel certain beyond any doubt. The problem is how to establish when you are certain. You may be clear when you feel happy or angry, but certain? Generally, if you think about whether you are 100% certain about almost anything, if you really search yourself, a doubt will most likely cross your mind, however small. So if you are busy with checking, you may have experienced doubts such as: what if I was checking on autopilot and actually did not do it properly; what if I can't trust my senses? What if I was momentarily distracted by a thought about something else? This can happen very frequently if you have a series of checks to perform. The logical response to a doubt like this is to go back and check again, which in turn can lead to more doubt. Therefore the inevitable experience of having doubts when checking means that it is often a long time before you will feel 100% *certain* that things are safe. An added problem is that you will probably feel anxious while doing the checks. By definition, anxiety is associated with feeling unsafe and uncertain because the stakes are high. We all feel more doubt when we are anxious because it is so important to get things right. Remember the example of *Who Wants To Be A Millionaire?* on page 71 – the more you question or doubt yourself, the less certain you become.

---

**CASE EXAMPLE**

*Jennifer had always been a careful person by nature. When she went to university in a town away from home, she moved into a flat with other students in her second year. Early in the term, Jennifer read a news story about a fire in some student flats in which a young person had died. Following this, Jennifer found that after her flatmates rushed out in the morning, she would carefully go round the house and check sockets and appliances such as the oven and hair straighteners in case anything that could cause a fire had been left on. She would check each item several times as it was easy to forget whether or not she had checked something as she went round. If she was going to the trouble of checking she wanted to make sure she had done it properly. She felt intensely anxious as she went about the house checking things. This would last until she got out of the house and absorbed into activities at university.*

*Although she was a very careful person, this was because deep down Jennifer had a suspicion that really she was someone prone to making mistakes. When she lived with friends Jennifer was responsible for herself for the first time. She became more aware of the possible danger that might be caused by her not taking care. This was brought into focus by reading a news story about a*

---

> fire and its terrible cost to life. Jennifer held the belief that
> if she did not act when she foresaw danger, then she was
> to blame for it if it happened. After reading the article,
> when she had the thought 'Did I leave something on?', she
> felt that it was really very little effort to go and check, given
> that the consequences of not checking could be so severe.
> She lived by the maxim 'better safe than sorry'.

## HOW DOES A CHECKING PROBLEM GET WORSE?

### Feeding into negative beliefs

We have seen how the act of checking can increase doubt and anxiety. It can also undermine people's confidence in themselves and can therefore seem to confirm beliefs that they hold about being careless. Research shows that people who check obsessively consistently rate their memories as poor. It makes sense, then, that this contributes to their checking as they feel that they may be a liability if they stop doing it. However, when their memories were actually tested there was no difference between people who did and did not have a checking problem.

### Selective attention

We all filter out irrelevant information from our environment. Checking focuses your attention on danger and therefore increases the amount of worries and doubts you experience. If we are in threat mode, we notice things which are consistent with this. Checking can make you go 'looking for trouble' (see page 75 for more on this); the more you check, the more you notice things which need checking which may not have troubled you before.

### Reassurance-seeking

Asking others for reassurance is itself a form of check. If you do this repeatedly, that should itself tell you that it doesn't really work. This is because, again, if the aim is to feel completely certain about something then you will always find a reason not to trust the answer. Perhaps they just wanted you to feel better? Perhaps they weren't sure themselves? As with other forms of checking, reassurance increases doubt. A further problem with this is that it has an impact on relationships. Being asked the same question repeatedly can be draining, and answers may become less sincere, further fuelling the problem of doubt.

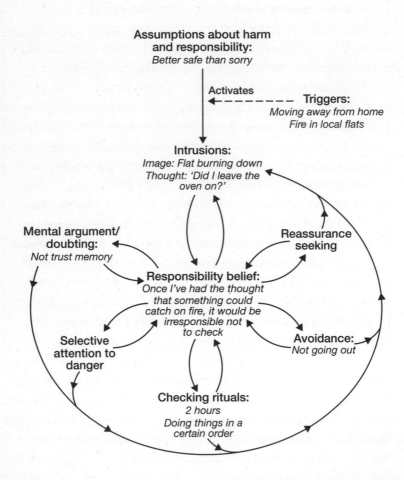

*Gradually, the amount of time Jennifer spent checking and the number of different things she checked increased. Jennifer now spent two hours each morning trying to leave the house. She developed a particular order in which she would check to try to be certain that she had been careful enough and checked everything. If her mind wandered from the task, or she felt uncertain, she would have to go back to the beginning of the list and start again. She often tried to visualise the things she checked in order to remember whether she had made them safe. She thought about the house a lot in the day and would sometimes have to hurry back home if she thought that she had missed something. Her flatmates would try to reassure her that the house was safe but this was never enough for Jennifer.*

*Once Jennifer had got into a pattern of checking, she was in a state of red alert and very focused on possible dangers in the house. However, the more she thought about it, the more things it occurred to her she should check if she was going to do the job properly. Her solution to this was to find ways to check more thoroughly. This had the effect of increasing the focus on danger. But it also set up a very high standard for the checking she needed to be completely sure that things were safe before she could move on.*

## WHAT HAPPENS IF THE OCD CARRIES ON GROWING?
### Avoidance

Once a checking problem gets worse, it can begin to interfere with many parts of life and even to take over. You may find that it is taking so long to leave the house that you are arranging things around the problem, going to things late. You may think that on some days it just isn't worth going out at all. Although you may reduce the amount of time checking, you are not free and able to do what you want. Avoidance keeps the problem going as the beliefs underlying the problem remain unchallenged. For example 'I cannot leave the house without checking'.

Avoidance means that the problem has not gone away, but has been accommodated into your life. In this way, OCD can be very destructive.

> *Jennifer soon found that she was frequently late for her lectures in the morning, and when she did attend, that she was thinking about her morning checking routine. After a while it became easier to arrange to do things in the afternoon only. She felt very ashamed, but managed to organise things around her worries. However, as she would still have to do several hours of checking in order to leave the house, it soon felt safer and much easier to stay in for most of the day. When people visited, Jennifer would feel extremely worried about whether they had inadvertently turned something on that she had turned off and would perform her checks after they left.*
>
> *Jennifer began to rearrange her life around the problem, fuelling the idea that the checks were working well by keeping her from making a mistake. She found that even though she did not go out herself, there were still things to worry about within the house. Her style of thinking and worries about danger became far more of a problem than any actual danger.*

## SUMMARY

A checking problem arises from reasonable concerns, but over time the checking becomes more of a problem than the thing you fear. It should be clear that the things you do because of those fears actually serve to make the checking problem worse. This works on two different levels. The behaviours keep you anxious and focused on danger, but they also stop you finding out what would happen if you didn't do the check.

| SAFETY-SEEKING BEHAVIOUR | HOW IT KEEPS THE PROBLEM GOING |
|---|---|
| Checking things repeatedly | Keeps focus on danger and increases doubt. Undermines confidence in memory. Keeps you feeling anxious |
| Asking for reassurance | Reassurance is a form of checking – it makes you feel less certain as you will always be able to pick holes in someone's answer |
| Avoidance | Avoidance means that the beliefs remain unchallenged. For example 'I cannot leave the house without checking' |

| ANXIETY-RELATED BELIEF | HOW IT KEEPS THE PROBLEM GOING |
|---|---|
| 'Once I've thought that something could go on fire, it would be irresponsible not to check' | To check is to be focused on danger. If you are checking, you will have more and more thoughts about danger. If you have to act on each one, you will soon find yourself doing lots more checking, thinking about more and more danger, doing more checking |
| 'I have a very poor memory' | Research shows that people with OCD do not have worse memories than others. However, doing lots of checking makes people less confident about their memory, a problem that they solve by ... doing more checking! |
| 'I can't stop checking until I feel certain that things are safe' | Feelings are not a good way to make decisions like this. Checking makes you feel anxious, and anxiety makes you doubt and feel uncertain. Therefore it's easy to get stuck in a loop of trying to feel certain by checking, which makes you feel less certain, so checking more |
| Nothing bad has happened – the checking is working to keep me and others safe | This is very seductive logic. But perhaps the checking is **nothing to do** with the fact that nothing bad has happened |

# CONTAMINATION/WASHING OCD

Most of us are brought up to be aware of dirt and germs and get into helpful habits of washing our hands after using the toilet or before eating food. As children we are told to not touch things that are 'dirty' (such as the inside of a rubbish bin or dog faeces) and are warned against 'spreading germs' by sneezing or coughing. As adults we generally keep up these habits as they are helpful in protecting us against communicable diseases such as stomach bugs or colds, and from food poisoning.

Many people have short periods of time when they become more concerned with disease. From time to time there is a lot of information in the media telling us to wash our hands to avoid spreading disease (such as swine flu) or to avoid food poisoning. If someone in your household is ill with flu or diarrhoea then it is sensible to wash your hands after touching them or using the toilet. We have all had times when we have been on a bus and touched something slimy and wanted to wash our hands straight away when we got home. Maybe when cooking for other people we might worry about salmonella and be more cautious than usual. You may have had occasions when your hands were visibly covered in something unpleasant – you may have come into contact with faeces, blood or an unknown sticky substance – and you probably washed your hands at the earliest opportunity.

As occasional worries, these things are not a problem. It is normal to want to wash your hands on such occasions, then to carry on doing your usual activities. Even if you prefer to wash your hands after, for example, using public transport, so long as you don't absolutely *have to*, this is not an obsessive problem. So if you can usually think 'I'd like to wash my hands before eating this sandwich, but I can't – I'm going to eat it anyway' then this is not a problem for you.

However, if you find that you are very preoccupied with dirt and germs every day, worrying that most everyday objects are 'contaminated' with disease, this would lead to you washing your hands repeatedly and in such a way that exceeds what most people do to avoid disease. In contamination OCD, washing rarely provides anything other than temporary relief from the fear of contamination.

With contamination/washing OCD, it is very difficult to feel as if things are clean after washing them following contact with something 'dirty'. It might feel easier to go to great lengths to avoid contact with things that might be dirty. Hand-washing may be repeated and ritualised, taking several hours. This is, of course, what is called 'compulsive washing'. Similar washing rules might apply for other bits of the body, clothes, possessions or home involving large volumes of anti-bacterial soap or other cleaning products such as bleach. It might feel important to 'keep track' of what objects are 'clean' or 'dirty'.

In contamination OCD, it becomes impossible not to carry out repeated hand-washing, etc., as it feels like too big a risk to take. As with other obsessional concerns, the exact worries that bother people are varied and individual.

| EXAMPLES OF CONTAMINATION PROBLEMS | ANXIETY-RELATED BELIEF |
| --- | --- |
| Avoiding public toilets | People with AIDS have used this toilet; I will come into contact with their bodily fluids and contract HIV |
| Washing hands after using public transport | Someone may not have washed their hands after using the toilet or touching themselves intimately; this will transfer on to me which is disgusting and could make me ill |
| Always over-cooking food | If this is not properly cooked then I will/ other people will get food poisoning, become ill and die |
| Never making anyone at work a cup of tea | I might get germs in the cup and make them ill and they will blame me |

## Do you have a problem with contamination and compulsive washing?

Contamination concerns with compulsive washing are a very common form of OCD. Compulsive washing may be a problem for you if you do all or some of the following:

- Wash your hands over 20 times a day
- Wash your hands for over a minute each time you wash them
- Follow a strict and thorough pattern of hand-washing, covering every surface of your hands and wrists/forearms
- Use several bars of soap a week or use bleach or other cleaning products on your skin
- Wash your hands so much that your hands are red and sore
- Avoid washing because you know that if you start washing you can't stop
- Wash your hands because you feel contaminated by ideas, people or places which are connected in your mind to contamination ('mental contamination')

Most people wash their hands after going to the toilet, before eating, when preparing food and when their hands are visibly dirty (for example after gardening or changing the oil in the car). If you regularly wash your hands on other occasions then compulsive washing may be a problem for you. For example:

- Touching door handles
- Touching letters received in the post
- Using public transport
- Shaking hands with other people
- Putting away shopping
- Touching things which are linked in your mind to bad experiences or people

Not surprisingly, once you start washing your hands a lot you might want to avoid situations that you consider dirty. This might include:

- Avoiding public transport
- Wearing gloves or using your sleeve to touch things when out
- Avoid picnics, going to the beach or parks
- Avoiding leaving the house altogether

Do you worry about something bad happening if you don't wash your hands, such as:

- Contracting HIV, TB, swine flu or other diseases?
- Spreading disease to others?
- Having a 'contaminated' feeling that you can't get rid of ?

---

**DO I HAVE CONTAMINATION/WASHING OCD?**
- Are you preoccupied by dirt/germs/disease?
- Do you feel very anxious until you wash your hands?
- Do you worry that something bad will happen if you don't wash your hands?
- Do you avoid many people/places/activities as you consider them dirty?

---

## HOW DOES CONTAMINATION/WASHING OCD BECOME A PROBLEM?

*Background experiences/ideas and trigger events*

As with other forms of OCD, beliefs we hold about ourselves, other people and the world around us can be involved in the development of contamination/washing OCD. It could be that people with contamination worries are concerned that others would blame them or think very badly of them if they did something such as give someone food poisoning. Some people with contamination concerns may have had a bad experience with a disease or someone close to them may have been very ill or died. However, we know that not everyone who has these background beliefs or experiences goes on to develop contamination OCD, so this is only part of the picture. For a lot of people there is no obvious reason why these problems arise. Sometimes the problem gets very gradually worse over a number of years, making it difficult to identify a particular point when the problem began.

## THE MEANING OF THE THOUGHTS/ANXIETY BELIEFS

If you are someone who worries a great deal about contamination, it is likely that when you have a thought 'What is that on my hand?' or 'What if this chicken has salmonella?' or a doubt such as 'Did I wash my hands properly after using the loo?' you find it difficult to ignore or dismiss. Believing that you need to do something to avoid potential harm (from disease) means that you treat these thoughts as important or significant and do something to try to prevent something bad happening. The problem is that while it is possible that something is dirty, that doesn't actually mean that it will definitely cause disease or that it is your responsibility to do anything about it. The inflated sense of responsibility that you feel for preventing harm leads to the lengthy washing, which in turn makes it feel like it is important to keep paying attention to dirt or germs to prevent something bad happening and to try to feel less anxious.

---

**CASE EXAMPLE**

*Suse read a lot of magazines with 'true life' stories about people recovering from life-threatening diseases. She noticed that a lot of people in the stories had picked up infections or diseases such as MRSA or salmonella. She started paying more attention to how clean things were in*

---

> her home, buying anti-bacterial spray and making sure
> that she was very careful when preparing food. When she
> was cooking, she would often think 'What if that had raw
> meat on it?' or 'What if that has salmonella?' and would
> throw the food away.

Suse was a sensible person who didn't like taking risks in life. She was also a very sensitive and considerate person, and felt very upset when she heard about bad things happening to other people. After reading so many horrible stories, Suse had started to feel very responsible for preventing the spread of any potential contamination or disease. Despite never having contracted a disease in her life so far, she started to feel extremely concerned that it was likely that this would happen and thought about how awful it would be. The idea of a disease or any bodily fluid being on her hands had become extremely frightening, due to the idea that she could die or, what might be even worse, pass the disease on to someone else who would become ill and die.

## HOW DOES A CONTAMINATION/WASHING PROBLEM GET WORSE?
### Why take the risk? Paying a high price
Washing your hands might feel like a small price to pay to avoid the risk of something terrible happening. However, when you think about the disruption caused to your life (and probably to other people's lives) and the time taken up, is it really a small price? What have you stopped doing, or stopped enjoying because of these concerns? Many people stop going out, stop touching other people, avoid many foods due to these concerns. Most importantly, how do you feel when you are paying this price? Does washing your hands really make you feel better and less anxious? Does it make the idea that something bad will happen go away? Or does it actually keep these ideas around, keep you feeling anxious and

miserable and stop you doing what you need or want to do? What is more, you don't get to find out what would happen if you don't wash your hands – that actually people are unlikely to get ill or die.

## Keeping track of dirt/germs – impossible criteria

If you think that an object is contaminated with dirt or germs, it is tempting to put that object 'in isolation' until you can clean it or dispose of it. The problem with this is, firstly, that you are treating your thoughts or doubts about contamination as true, which makes them feel more important. Secondly, it is very difficult to keep track of what is 'dirty' and what is not without devoting a great deal of time and attention to the task – which means that you can't do other things that you need or want to do, and you end up preoccupied and anxious.

## 'Feeling right' – impossible criteria

If you hold the frightening belief that something bad will happen if you don't wash your hands, it would follow that you now wash your hands in a very thorough, ritualised way to try to be certain that you have removed all possible contamination. If you don't do it in this way, it may not 'feel right' – this is not surprising, given you have got into the habit of doing it in this particular way. However, using 'feeling right' to judge how to wash your hands generally leads to hand-washes becoming longer, more intricate and more rigid to try to fulfil that 'impossible criterion'. In turn this makes you feel more anxious, and more focused on your belief that it is important to worry about contamination (see page 62 which describes how this works in more detail).

> Suse washed her hands 50 times a day, spending two to three minutes doing a 'surgical scrub' where she focused on every surface of her hand and wrist. She would do this thorough hand-wash after going to the toilet and while she

was cooking, but also after touching anything that some-one else could have touched. This included door handles, the 'stop' button on public transport, items in the super-market and her post. She would notice small red or brown marks on objects and think 'that could be blood or faeces' and throw them out. She would feel extremely anxious until she was able to wash her hands; when she was out of the house she would use alcohol rub and wet wipes to clean her hands. Her hands were red raw and swollen, frequently cracked and bleeding. Despite this, she would often wash her hands again as they didn't 'feel' clean.

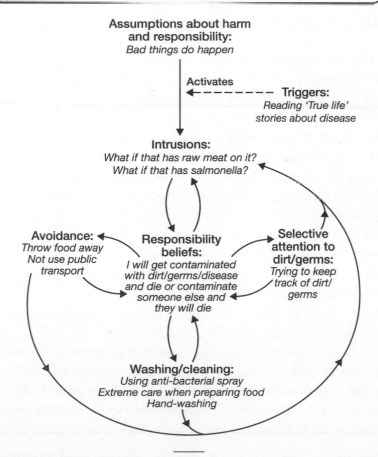

Assumptions about harm and responsibility:
*Bad things do happen*

Activates

Triggers:
*Reading 'True life' stories about disease*

Intrusions:
*What if that has raw meat on it? What if that has salmonella?*

Avoidance:
*Throw food away Not use public transport*

Responsibility beliefs:
*I will get contaminated with dirt/germs/disease and die or contaminate someone else and they will die*

Selective attention to dirt/germs:
*Trying to keep track of dirt/germs*

Washing/cleaning:
*Using anti-bacterial spray Extreme care when preparing food Hand-washing*

## What happens if the OCD carries on growing?

### Avoidance

Many people with obsessional beliefs about contamination start to avoid numerous situations as it feels easier and less anxiety-provoking to not have any contact that might involve dirt or germs. This could mean not using public transport, not touching other people or not leaving the house at all. Clearly this has a hugely negative effect on the ability to function in the world.

### More extreme and extensive rituals

As OCD becomes more severe, it feels more believable that something terrible will happen. This can lead to devastatingly long and complex rituals – such as taking eight hours to have a shower. Sometimes people dread the lengthy rituals so much that they actually avoid doing them – so it is not uncommon for the paradoxical situation to arise when someone with a fear of dirt and germs actually avoids having a shower for weeks or months as they know it will take so long to do it 'properly'.

### But this isn't how it works for me ...

If you wash your hands a great deal but don't have any contamination concerns similar to the examples given here, there are several other things to consider:

### 'Mental contamination'

The most common reason why people compulsively wash their hands is to avoid contact with dirt, germs/disease and other forms of 'contamination'. However, sometimes people wash their hands to try to remove a 'dirty' feeling associated with a particular person or horrible experience. OCD still works in the same way; engaging in rituals or avoidance will only temporarily remove this feeling, and perpetuates the anxiety. On page 95, the way this works is described in greater detail. An important step in dealing with mental contamination is seeing it for what it is ... often, this is about feeling dirty because you have been 'treated like dirt', betrayed or otherwise treated badly by people you trusted. It is understandable that people who feel contaminated by awful things done to them want to wash away their feelings of being violated, but of course this doesn't really work ... you can't wash away what's inside your head (although it might seem that washing makes you feel better for a short time). Once the person is able to recognise that the washing does not help with the real problem, this opens the way to refocusing on the real problem. Often this will require expert and specialist help in order to begin to come to terms with the things which made the person feel dirty in the first place. See also page 237 for further discussion of how to deal with OCD linked to traumatic experiences.

**'I know I won't get a disease, but I don't want to lose track of the contamination – I'll feel out of control.'**
In Chapter 5 we will spend a lot of time on the questions 'What is so bad about that?' and 'What's the worst thing that could happen?' So even if you are not worried about disease, there will be something that is anxiety provoking about 'losing track' of the contamination or feeling 'out of control'.

**'Other people *are* dirty – I've got it right to be this careful about dirt and germs.'**
If it really doesn't bother you, or interfere in your life to take extensive precautions to avoid contamination, then OCD is not a problem for you. However, if when you think about it, you are paying a high price to avoid the risk in terms of hours spent washing or cleaning, avoiding other people, giving up on enjoyable activities, being preoccupied with thoughts about dirt and germs – then it is worth considering taking the 'risk' of doing things differently. We can never guarantee that nothing bad will happen, but we can guarantee that OCD will get worse and take over your life if you continue to avoid and engage in safety-seeking behaviours.

**THE INSURANCE POLICIES**

An insurance salesperson comes to your door.

'I have two policies on sale today. The first covers you for fire, flood, accidental damage and theft; it's £50 a month. The second, de luxe policy, covers you for fire, flood, accidental damage, theft, alien invasion, plague, meteor strike and Acts of God. This is a million pounds a month. Which policy would you prefer?'

'Well, I'll have the first one.'

'But the second one is much more comprehensive – these things might well happen – surely you want to insure against that risk?'

'But I can't afford one million pounds a month – the price is too high – these things might happen, and they would be awful, but they are not that likely. If I spend any more than £50 a month I would have to go without something else that I need or want.'

Although it is not obvious at first, OCD works this way. Don't take risks, it says. Better safe than sorry. What only becomes obvious much later in OCD is the true cost of avoiding any possible risk. OCD takes over everything in your life, your happiness, your relationships, takes all your free time and so on. The things OCD takes away from you are priceless, and you actually get no protection at all. You also get all kinds of real harm. OCD is a sleazy insurance salesman!

## SUMMARY

If you believe that you are responsible for preventing something bad happening, such as spreading disease, you will feel very anxious and do things to try to lower the risk of that happening. All the things you do actually have the effect of refocusing you on your belief that something bad will happen and make you feel more anxious. They can lead to tragic consequences such as never leaving the house or touching anyone else.

| ANXIETY-RELATED BELIEF | HOW IT KEEPS THE PROBLEM GOING |
|---|---|
| I am responsible for preventing the spread of contamination/dirt/germs and stopping something bad happening – illness or death | No one can actually stop the spread of all dirt/germs/disease. All your efforts to try to reduce the risk actually focus on the potential danger and lead to you feeling more responsible, not less |
| If there is any risk that something is dirty/contaminated, I must do something about it | By not taking the risk, you don't get to find out that actually nothing bad happens |

| SAFETY-SEEKING BEHAVIOUR | HOW IT KEEPS THE PROBLEM GOING |
|---|---|
| Washing hands or other body parts or inanimate objects in a repetitive, ritualised way | Once lengthy washing starts, any shorter or less comprehensive washing doesn't feel 'enough'. Rituals and repeating don't make things any cleaner; the only result is feeling more anxious |
| Using how your hands 'feel' to work out when to stop washing | This is a dangerous way to decide to stop washing; the more anxious you feel, the more you feel dirty, the more you wash, the more anxious you feel ... |
| Avoiding touching, e.g. door handles | By avoiding, you prevent yourself from finding out what would happen if you do touch all these things – that actually you are unlikely to contract a disease or spread it to anyone else |

| | |
|---|---|
| Being on the 'lookout for trouble', e.g. looking for red or brown marks, (blood or faeces) monitoring yourself or other people for signs of ill health | This is a form of selective attention; once you start looking, you will spot marks on objects that no one else would have seen. By throwing the objects out ('better safe than sorry') you do not have the opportunity to find out that the marks on the objects were harmless. By tuning in to whether anyone is showing signs of ill health, you will notice the smallest sniff or cough |

## RUMINATION OCD

Throughout the day we have all sorts of thoughts going through our minds, whether we are conscious of this or not. The content of thoughts could be anything. Thoughts may come into our minds prompted by some cue, such as seeing a card shop and remembering that it is a friend's birthday. At other times thoughts can be unprompted, seeming to 'pop in' from nowhere. In the case of a thought about say, picking up the dry-cleaning, a memory of a great holiday or getting a fantastic idea for a story, the sudden appearance of these thoughts is unlikely to be troublesome and we will probably think of them as useful, positive or just neutral thoughts and may even forget about them seconds later. However, given the nature of our minds, eventually we are bound to think of something that could be considered negative, such as thinking about a relative dying or thinking how easy it might be to jump in front of the next train. For some people, experiencing such negative 'intrusive thoughts' can be very uncomfortable as they wonder *why* they had that thought and what it means about them to have it.

Obsessive rumination describes the process of reacting to upsetting intrusive thoughts by thinking about them over again and again in an attempt to resolve this discomfort. This type of OCD *looks* different from other forms in that there are no obvious physical compulsions, and it is sometimes referred to as 'pure O' to reflect this. However, although they may not be obvious, the compulsions are going on inside the person's mind. They may take the form of 'cancelling out' the worrying thought with other thoughts, or mentally 'wrestling' or arguing with it. Sometimes there are also a number of very subtle physical compulsions such as avoidance of particular situations and generally taking extra care with things, depending on the content of the rumination. Sometimes obsessional rumination can occur along with overt physical compulsions.

| INTRUSIVE THOUGHT | CONTENT OF RUMINATIONS |
|---|---|
| A heterosexual person having an image of someone of the same sex when having a sexual experience | Am I gay? |
| Thinking that a schoolchild is pretty | Am I a paedophile? |
| Thought about death | Is this a premonition? |
| Thinking how easy it would be to drown your baby when bathing them | Could I just go mad and do something terrible? |
| My thoughts don't fit with OCD | What if I don't have OCD and am actually a terrible person for having negative thoughts? |

There may be times when most people would respond to an intrusive thought like the ones above by wondering what it meant about them. In rumination OCD the person is really stuck in the doubt and cannot move on without trying to mentally resolve the worry. You can identify whether or not your responses to thoughts are compulsions by asking yourself, when

I get my troubling intrusive thought, can I just let it go and dismiss it without feeling too worried? If the answer is no, and you find that you are spending a lot of time in repetitive, circular, anxiety-provoking thinking about the meaning of your thoughts and why you are having them, then you may have the rumination type of OCD.

## RUMINATION IS NOT RANDOM!

For many people troubled by constant rumination, the question 'Why am I having this thought?' is really important. And the reality is that rumination is not random. There is a pattern; loving mothers and fathers are troubled by thoughts of harming, abusing or neglecting their children, the religious person is troubled by blasphemous thoughts, the gentle person by thoughts of violence, the open-minded person by racist thoughts and so on. So what does this pattern mean? Well, it means that in OCD the intrusive thoughts focus on *your worst fears*. What could be worse (and more upsetting) for the loving mother than the idea and image of sticking a needle in her baby's eye? Having had that thought, you might recognise it for what it is (your worst fear), and you would shudder and get on with feeding your much-loved baby. However, some people are (understandably) so horrified by the idea which has intruded into their mind that they jump to the wrong conclusion ... 'Having this thought means that I'm a sick pervert, a child abuser'. This misinterpretation can and does, in OCD, lead to a whole bunch of problematic reactions ... backing away from baby, insisting that others be with you whenever you are with baby, trying to push the thoughts out of your mind and all the other counterproductive, obsessional reactions described above. Not to mention the unbearable fear and unhappiness that follows this interpretation ... which, of course, makes your thinking patterns even more negative, in one of those vicious circles which makes OCD thrive. See also page 77.

**DO I HAVE RUMINATION OCD?**

Have you had thoughts, doubts or images that you find upsetting or think that you shouldn't have? When your thoughts are bothering you, do you:

- Try to work out what your thoughts mean?
- Push the thoughts out of your head or try to deliberately think about something 'good'?
- Try to argue with the thoughts or yourself?
- Try to seek reassurance from others that the thoughts don't mean what you think they do?
- Do you mentally review your thoughts and/or actions over and over again?
- Does this process make you feel anxious?
- Do you spend significant amounts of time doing this, at the cost of other things in life?

## WHEN IS IT NOT OCD?

Rumination is a psychological process that accompanies many different disorders. For example, in depression, people commonly ruminate about why things went wrong for them, or why they are so worthless. This type of rumination tends to focus on past events and keeps the person's mood very low. In everyday life, rumination accompanies everyday stress. Mulling things over may help us to work out how to progress with certain problems. However, taken to a clinical level, unhelpful rumination or worry is part of a problem known as generalised anxiety disorder (GAD), in which worries about everyday matters take over the person's life. People with GAD are constantly worrying about all sorts of disasters and pitfalls that may or may not happen, for example, 'What if I can't pay my next gas bill?' or 'What if my husband leaves me?' The worry dominates to the extent that they cannot enjoy the positive things in life. They often begin to worry about the fact that they are worrying and this becomes a vicious circle.

Rumination in OCD differs in that the anxiety is caused by the actual experience of having the negative thought in the first place rather than worrying too much about a number of everyday topics. The anxiety stems from the feeling that having such a thought seems to signify something bad about you and that you need to deal with the thought by thinking more about it.

## HOW DOES RUMINATION BECOME A PROBLEM?
### Background beliefs and trigger events
As with all forms of OCD, people with ruminations are often very careful and conscientious by nature. Increases in stress and levels of responsibility may contribute to rumination in a general sense. In some cases, the onset is a clear experience of a particular negative thought in a certain context that filled the person with anxiety and dread.

Rumination describes a style of responding to intrusive thoughts – the content can be very varied, entirely individual and can also change over time for the same person. What is always true is that they find the thoughts they are having troublesome and anxiety provoking. The reason that intrusive thoughts bother an individual is because, for them, the thought could indicate that something is true about them that they find particularly abhorrent. What this means varies from person to person. For example a new mother may be horrified by an intrusive thought of smothering her child as it could mean that she is a terrible person capable of something awful. In rumination OCD the person gets absorbed into trying to understand the content of the thoughts and what it means to have the thought in the first place.

### The meaning of thoughts
In combination with general background circumstances, specific beliefs about the nature and importance of thoughts are very important in the development of rumination OCD. It is common to believe that 'if I think something bad it is the same as doing something bad' and 'if I have a thought I must want it to happen'.

Beliefs also play an important role in how people then respond to disturbing thoughts. Frequent examples are 'it is wrong to ignore thoughts' and 'I cannot take the risk of the thought coming true'.

## Mental argument and the need for certainty

Rumination often includes grappling with the meaning of the thought to try to decide whether or not it is true. As the interpretation is often very frightening for the person (am I bad/mad/perverted?), understandably they frequently want to be absolutely sure that they are not what they fear before moving on – the 'argument' needs to be settled. The difficulty here is that the argument is futile because the intrusive thought or doubt is just random mental junk; engaging in mental argument makes the thought feel more important and believable.

For many things that are the focus of obsessive ruminations, it is hard to be completely certain that they are not true. How can you *prove* to yourself beyond any doubt that you are a good person? We can probably all think of an example where we acted impulsively, offended someone or otherwise did something wrong, or had what might be a sexual thought that didn't fit with our sexual orientation. Does this mean that we are bad, or somehow lying to ourselves? In reality, these sorts of characteristics are more complex than that; shades of grey rather than black and white – just because you can think of an example of not being 100% good does not mean that you are 100% bad. So if you think about whether you are 100% certain about these types of attributes, if you really search yourself, a doubt will most likely cross your mind, however small. This is particularly difficult if you need to be certain before you can allow yourself to move on and stop thinking about something. In fact, the more you try to be certain, the less certain you feel. In this way, people can get stuck in loops of rumination.

In rumination OCD, the person gets absorbed into trying to understand the content of the thoughts. However, the process that primarily keeps the problem going is the rumination itself.

## CASE EXAMPLE

*Jeremy became a parent for the first time in his early thirties. He had always thought of himself as a responsible person and was looking forward to the birth of his child. He and his partner were thrilled when the little girl arrived and were very careful and loving parents. When the baby was six weeks old, Jeremy was changing her nappy when he had the thought 'You might die'. Jeremy was instantly filled with a feeling of dread and wondered why this thought had come into his mind at this point. The anxiety was so strong that he had a terrible fear that this could mean that, even though it was the last thing he wanted, perhaps somewhere deep down he had negative thoughts about his own child. Although he wasn't particularly superstitious about other things, this felt too important to ignore. He had read newspaper stories about men killing their children and worried about falling into that state of mind, whatever it was. He said carefully to himself 'I don't want you to die; I'll keep you safe'. He then had a worry that these were just words and that he did not really mean them. Jeremy began to look for evidence that he loved the baby and did not want anything bad to happen to her.*

*Jeremy experienced a negative intrusive thought at a time when he felt happy and was looking after his vulnerable new baby. As the thought was completely unexpected and did not fit with the situation, it 'stood out' in his thinking which made it feel important. Jeremy's first reaction was that it actually meant that something dreadful would happen. His beliefs about the importance of thoughts made his unexpectedly negative thought very difficult to ignore. As he struggled to understand the thought, he felt mounting anxiety about his own feelings towards the baby and with each attempt to reassure himself, he felt more doubt. As his anxiety rose, he felt more afraid that he was going to lose control.*

## How does a rumination problem get worse?

### Anxiety as evidence

A common pitfall in OCD is to think that 'because I feel anxious there must be something wrong'. This is particularly toxic, as the meaning given to the thought causes anxiety, which is then taken as evidence that the interpretation was correct. This is circular reasoning, but can be very powerful when you are stuck in a pattern of rumination. If something 'feels' true, this does not make it true, although it seems a part of human nature to give credibility to these feelings. Many a gambler has fallen foul of 'feeling' lucky when they placed their bet which lost them everything.

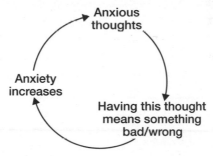

### 'Magical' thinking

Superstitions are common to all societies. The specifics vary immensely from putting shoes on a table to walking under a ladder or breaking a mirror. In each case, going against the superstition will somehow cause something bad to happen eventually. There is no mechanism by which these things can cause 'bad luck', so it is by some sort of 'magic' that this happens. The ideas are so ingrained within society that it is common to feel dread or anxiety when you break a superstition, even if you consider yourself a very rational person. In the course of life, sooner or later any given person will have something bad happen to them, or to someone they love and it is common to attribute this to bringing bad luck on yourself by having broken a superstitious belief. Needless to say many good things will happen in the same time period but these are readily ignored. This sort of general and non-specific association fuels the idea that going against the superstition some-how caused the bad thing to happen. Magical thinking can play a role in rumination problems by the coincidence of events that leads to someone assuming a causal link.

### The meaning of mental argument

Rumination, the going over of thoughts and events, increases doubt and anxiety. Because of this it can also undermine people's confidence in themselves and can therefore seem to support their beliefs about being bad or dangerous. A further problem is that sometimes people develop an additional belief that they may be going mad *because* they are ruminating for hours. In these terms if they 'accept the thoughts' and stop ruminating they are bad and if they stay stuck in OCD they feel like they are crazy. This is a very tangled OCD web.

> *Jeremy became ultra-careful when doing anything for the baby, especially when he was changing her nappy. He would approach this task with trepidation and could feel himself getting anxious as the time approached in case he had a 'bad' thought. He would always say to himself before doing this that he loved the baby very much and that he did not want her to die. He would list the reasons for this to himself – that he looked after the baby, that he had wanted the baby. Yet sometimes when he looked at the baby he found it very difficult to be certain that he was feeling 'complete' love. He wondered if he was kidding himself, that he was just playing a role. Maybe he was capable of doing something bad as he was having all of these crazy thoughts. He did not talk about his intrusive thoughts but he asked for a lot of reassurance from friends and family that he was a nice person.*

The more Jeremy ruminated, the more anxious he felt, and the more he felt driven to ruminate in order to really understand whether or not he was dangerous. Trying to search himself for evidence he 'loved' his baby only made the problem worse as it was very difficult to define what he was looking for, and therefore impossible to actually find a definitive answer. This only made him feel more anxious and he got more intrusive thoughts that seemed to suggest the opposite.

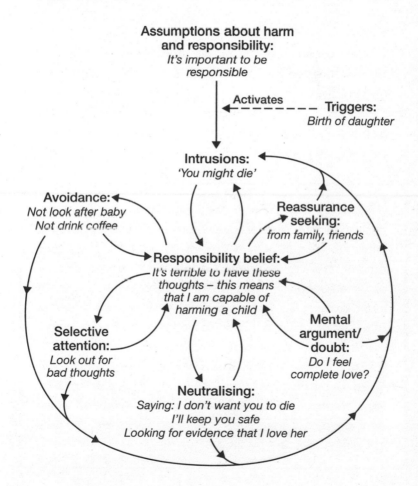

## WHAT HAPPENS IF THE OCD CARRIES ON GROWING?

Once rumination takes hold, it can begin to interfere with many parts of life and even to take over. You may find that it is taking a lot of time, and making it hard to be around people as your mind is so full of these thoughts. They are probably also keeping your mood very low. Sometimes you might feel anxious or resentful at others for interrupting your ruminations, or saying something that triggers a new set of rumination.

### Rumination: avoidance

Trying to keep yourself safe by avoiding 'dangerous' situations, means that the problem has not gone away, but has been accommodated into your life. This is a powerful way of fuelling the belief that you need to take special precautions to stay safe, that your worst fear is in fact true. Avoidance also means limiting your life in some way and can be very destructive.

> *Jeremy began to get more thoughts that he didn't love the baby and that he might want her to die. When he had these thoughts he would turn away from the baby and repeat 'I love you and I don't want you to die'. He felt very ashamed at having these thoughts. Soon Jeremy began to make excuses so that he did not have to look after the baby, much to the annoyance of his partner who wasn't aware of how serious his concerns were. He started to question himself in other areas of life, such as whether he loved his partner or had in fact loved his parents. He was very preoccupied for most of the time. Although other people may not have been able to tell, for Jeremy life was completely clouded by OCD.*

Jeremy was unable to resolve his doubts by mental argument and reassurance, so he began to change his life to fit around the OCD, just in case they were true. This began to have a huge effect on his mood and on those around him. His behaviour fuelled his belief that he was capable of something terrible as he acted as though this was true.

## SUMMARY

As with other forms of OCD, in rumination OCD it is how you interpret the fact you have negative thoughts that causes the anxiety. The compulsions come in the form of mental checks or arguments that attempt to prove that your interpretation was wrong.

| SAFETY-SEEKING BEHAVIOUR | HOW IT KEEPS THE PROBLEM GOING |
| --- | --- |
| Mentally reviewing events | This is a form of checking. It keeps focus on danger and increases doubt. Undermines confidence in memory. Keeps you feeling anxious |
| Thought suppression | Trying to suppress thoughts makes you have more of them. In order not to think of something, you need to think of what it is you are trying to push away |
| Asking for reassurance | Reassurance is a form of checking – it may give you temporary relief but ultimately makes you feel less certain as you will always be able to pick holes in the answer. |
| Avoidance | Avoidance means that the beliefs remain unchallenged; as you are 'acting as if' it is true, your obsessional belief feels more true |

| ANXIETY-RELATED BELIEF | HOW IT KEEPS THE PROBLEM GOING |
|---|---|
| Thinking something is as bad as doing it | This means that thoughts are themselves a source of danger – it is impossible to not have these thoughts |
| I am a bad and dangerous person or I wouldn't be having these thoughts | Because you are worried about being bad, you are on the lookout for 'bad thoughts'. Therefore you will notice every thought that fits with this idea and you will generate more of such thoughts. If this seems like 'evidence' then the belief will strengthen. This is a vicious circle |
| In order to feel safe, I need to be completely certain that I won't do something wrong | It is impossible to achieve a sense of certainty about obsessional doubts. The more you try to be certain, the less certain you will feel, and so you will get stuck in a vicious circle |
| The thoughts I have mean something fundamental about me | This belief will drive you to try to work out what the 'true' meaning of the thought is |
| Anxious thoughts can damage my brain | This is of course an anxiety-provoking thought and is an OCD trap |

# RELIGIOUS OCD (OR SCRUPULOSITY)

We know that the way OCD works is to interrupt and interfere with important bits of your life. If you are a religious person, OCD will try to infiltrate your religious life. Religious and moral obsessions are some of the earliest reported forms of OCD. Many famous religious figures in history have had disturbing intrusive thoughts and doubts about their faith; Martin Luther and John Bunyan are amongst the more famous.

'Blasphemous' thoughts are a very clear example of how the same thought can mean something different to different people. For example, a thought about a religious figure naked can be horrifying and upsetting to someone of that faith; it is insignificant to an atheist and may even be amusing to someone who feels strongly against religion.

It is a normal part of religious life to have doubts and questions about religious teachings, to question your faith or to feel concerned that you are not being observant or true to your faith. These doubts are something that people usually deal with by discussion or reflection, or the concerns pass. In religious OCD, these doubts will be repeated, disturbing and upsetting; they may be accompanied by disturbing images or thoughts about your religion. For many people affected, the OCD utterly overwhelms their true religious feelings.

If you have OCD about religion you will not be able to easily dismiss these thoughts or images; instead you have found yourself believing that these thoughts are significant and important. You may have felt very uncomfortable, anxious or disturbed by having the thoughts. You have probably found that the more you have paid attention to these thoughts, the harder it has been for you to actually follow and participate in your religion. You may have found yourself avoiding anything to do with your faith for fear of having intrusive thoughts, doubts or images. You may believe that these thoughts mean something very bad about you.

## DO YOU HAVE A PROBLEM WITH OCD ABOUT RELIGION?

- Have you had thoughts, doubts or images connected to your religion that you find upsetting or think that you shouldn't have?
- When you are praying or engaged in religious practice, are you frequently interrupted by upsetting thoughts, doubts or images?

If you are concerned about having these thoughts and believe that it might mean something bad about you, you might have started to try to do something about the thoughts, make amends for having them, or try to avoid having them in the first place. When these thoughts are bothering you, do you:

- Push the thoughts out of your head or try to deliberately think about something 'good'?
- Try to argue with the thoughts, or yourself?
- Pray more, perhaps using elaborate or repetitive prayers?
- Try to seek reassurance from others that you are religious enough or that you are not bad for having these thoughts?

Have you been avoiding:

- Going in, or even walking past, religious buildings?
- Touching or reading religious books or other items?
- Praying/observing religious practices?
- Mentioning these thoughts to anyone in your faith?

---

**DO I HAVE OCD ABOUT RELIGION?**
- Are you troubled by repeated intrusive thoughts, doubts or images connected to your religion?
- Have these thoughts led to you trying to stop having the thoughts and trying to make amends for having them?
- Have you been avoiding your religious practice?

---

## HOW DOES RELIGIOUS OCD BECOME A PROBLEM?
*Background experiences/ideas and trigger events*
It is possible to have OCD in any religion. It might be that if your religion is particularly rigid and strict there are more opportunities

to experience intrusive thoughts about whether you have behaved appropriately or carried out a religious practice properly. Sometimes people report having very 'black and white' interpretations of religion when they were young. For example, they may have been taught that God is all knowing and that sinners will be damned. Beliefs that can form that might be important in OCD include 'thinking something is as bad as doing it', 'it is wrong to think badly of anyone'.

### The meaning of thoughts/doubts/images; anxiety-related beliefs

In religious OCD, people believe that it is bad to have these thoughts, doubts or images, and that having these means that they are a bad person, which understandably leads to feeling anxious, guilty and upset. The problem with this belief is that we cannot control what we think – we all have intrusive thoughts about all manner of things. Intrusive religious thoughts are no different from other intrusive thoughts.

---

**CASE EXAMPLE**

*Johnson enjoyed going to church every week and studied his Bible every day. Once, when he was at home reading his Bible, he had an image of himself having sex with his best friend's girlfriend. He was upset that he had this thought at the time he was trying to concentrate on his Bible studies. His heart started racing and he became hot and flustered. He noticed tingling sensations in his genitals which upset him more.*

---

Johnson believed that people should be 'pure in thought, word and deed' and that 'thinking something is as bad as doing it'. For him, having this intrusive sexual thought was as bad as acting on the thought; having such a thought while reading his Bible meant that he was a bad person. This was confirmed for him by the feelings in his genitals which seemed to prove that it was not just a thought. Due to his belief that it was wrong to have these thoughts, he tried to do things to stop having them and to make sure that he wasn't becoming more 'sinful'.

## How does religious OCD get worse?

### Thought suppression

If you try not to think a particular thought, paradoxically the thought comes back more. Remember the 'white polar bears' example on page 72? If you try *not* to think about their cute babies and fluffy white faces … what most people find is that it is impossible not to picture polar bears. This works in the same way when you try not to have religious thoughts.

### Neutralising

Trying to confess, or make amends for, intrusive thoughts by praying buys into the idea that it is bad to have the thought in the first place. It refocuses your attention on the thoughts passing through your mind so that you will certainly notice any that could be 'wrong'. Furthermore, you will probably find that intrusive thoughts keep interrupting your prayers, which may make you feel that you need to start again or to pray more and more each time. It might be difficult to feel satisfied that your prayers are 'enough'.

### Mental argument

Trying to convince yourself or argue with yourself about whether you should have these thoughts or what they mean about you can lead to you feeling more preoccupied. It is unlikely that you will feel certain or reassure yourself by this process; mental argument is likely to make you feel more anxious.

## Rituals

It is common for prayers to take on a ritualised form, repeating certain phrases or having to say things a certain number of times. These ritualised prayers are unlikely to feel like your usual praying; the rituals will only give you temporary (if any) relief from anxiety.

## Selective attention

As you become more worried about your intrusive thoughts, you will start to notice the thoughts more. Similarly, if you are monitoring your body for sexual arousal, focusing on your genitals, you might assume that any sensation felt in that area is a sign of sexual arousal. Feeling anxious leads to many changes in bodily sensations; if you focus on *any* part of your body you will notice changes. Excitement and anxiety activate the same system.

## Reassurance

Seeking reassurance from other people is a very appealing strategy, as their replies may set your mind at rest for a short while. However, after a while more doubts might creep in, you may want to ask for more reassurance, ask the person if they are sure, explain again exactly what you mean to try to be certain that they are answering your question properly – you will require more and more reassurance to get any relief from your anxiety.

> Johnson tried to push the images out of his head; he found that the image became more explicit and he became more upset and anxious. He abandoned his reading and started to pray to ask for forgiveness for what he considered a sin. The next time Johnson went to church he was very worried that he would have sexual thoughts during the service. On his way to church he started to have thoughts about having sex with other members of the congregation and pictured the priest naked. He was very disturbed by these images

*and tried to think of Jesus and recite his favourite Bible passages. By the time he got to the church he was very anxious and felt sure that other people could tell that there was something wrong. He tried to work out whether he was getting sexually aroused and became aware of sensations in his genitals. He told his friends at church that he didn't feel well and went home. He felt ashamed and guilty for lying to his friends. He prayed for several hours but didn't dare read his Bible in case he had more thoughts.*

## WHAT HAPPENS IF THE OCD KEEPS GROWING?
### Avoidance

It can feel easier to avoid situations where having intrusive thoughts would feel worse. Avoiding your religious meetings or practice will probably make you feel more upset and guilty and make it feel more as if you are sinning and that you are a bad person. This can lead to further doubts about your commitment to your religion; these doubts might feel more true and believable as you actually spend less time engaged in your faith.

*Over the next week Johnson stayed away from his church friends, didn't read his Bible and devoted every evening to prayer. His prayers became more elaborate and time consuming and he found himself repeating certain phrases as he wasn't sure whether he was praying sincerely and genuinely. The more he repeated them, the less certain he felt that he was a good Christian. Johnson started having frequent doubts about whether he really was a Christian, and started to believe more that he was a bad or evil person.*

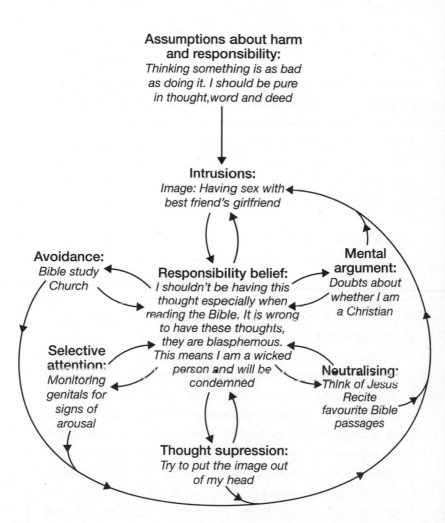

**Assumptions about harm and responsibility:**
*Thinking something is as bad as doing it. I should be pure in thought, word and deed*

**Intrusions:**
*Image: Having sex with best friend's girlfriend*

**Avoidance:**
*Bible study Church*

**Responsibility belief:**
*I shouldn't be having this thought especially when reading the Bible. It is wrong to have these thoughts, they are blasphemous. This means I am a wicked person and will be condemned*

**Mental argument:**
*Doubts about whether I am a Christian*

**Selective attention:**
*Monitoring genitals for signs of arousal*

**Neutralising:**
*Think of Jesus Recite favourite Bible passages*

**Thought supression:**
*Try to put the image out of my head*

*But this isn't how it works for me ...*

**I am not religious but I believe that thinking a bad thought
means I am a bad person**

For non-religious people, it is common to have doubts about
whether your behaviour is consistent to your personal moral
beliefs. This works in the same way as religious beliefs.

**How can I be certain that this is OCD and that it is
genuinely normal to have these thoughts – isn't religion
different from other thoughts?**

This is actually an example of an OCD doubt. Asking for help – not
reassurance – from your religious leader can be useful, if they are
someone you would turn to for help with other problems in your
life – this is no different.

You are likely to find that other people have spoken to them
about similar concerns, or that they may have had similar thoughts
or doubts themselves. They will want to help you to stop OCD
from interfering in your life. They will probably encourage you to
rejoin your religious group if you have been avoiding it – it will be
important to do this even if the thoughts are still bothering you.
They might suggest to you specific ways to gain strength from
your faith from prayer, or by doing active work in your community or from discussion with other members of your faith.

Occasionally, religious leaders may not be familiar with this
kind of problem; if so, try to speak to another person from your
faith. It is also helpful to speak to family members or friends who
you trust and who you consider to follow your religion in a similar way. If you are honest with them and let them know how
much this has been troubling you, you are likely to get their help
and support.

## SUMMARY

If you believe that it is wrong or bad to have certain thoughts or images, you will feel very anxious and try to do things to get the thoughts out of your head or to make amends. All the things you do actually keep the problem going by 'buying in' to the idea that these thoughts are important and significant and that you need to do something about them to stop yourself being a bad person. Something you can be completely clear about ... whichever God you believe in, it is quite clear that God would not want you to suffer from OCD, and would want you to do whatever you can to get rid of the OCD. Not to get rid of the intrusive thoughts (everyone has those, remember), but the OCD which interferes with your ability to freely practise your religion.

| ANXIETY-RELATED BELIEF | HOW IT KEEPS THE PROBLEM GOING |
|---|---|
| Having this thought means that I am a bad person | Your values and religious beliefs might mean that you are more likely to interpret an intrusive thought as significant and meaningful - but everyone has intrusive thoughts |
| I should be able to get rid of these thoughts | It is normal to have intrusive thoughts, images or doubts - it is impossible not to. Trying to get rid of the thoughts actually makes them more noticeable and treats the thoughts as important |

| SAFETY-SEEKING BEHAVIOUR | HOW IT KEEPS THE PROBLEM GOING |
|---|---|
| Trying not to think about it (thought suppression) | Suppressing thoughts actually generates more thoughts |
| Trying to think about something else (thought substitution) | This is 'buying in' to the idea that the thought is significant and wrong and that it is necessary to get rid of it by substituting another thought – the original thought is likely to come back again, and more |
| Selective attention – to thoughts or body parts | Being on the lookout for thoughts makes them more noticeable. Feeling anxious can lead to many changes in bodily sensations; by paying attention to his genitals, he guaranteed that he would notice some changes |
| Rituals – e.g. praying for hours to ask for forgiveness | Prayers become repetitive and prolonged and 'buy in' to the idea that it is wrong to have the thought in the first place. Trying to get the prayer 'right' can bring on more of the intrusive thoughts and images and fresh doubts about your faith |
| Avoiding religious practice | By avoiding activities that are consistent with observance of your faith you may feel more upset and guilty and your belief that you are bad can feel more believable and true |

## UNDERSTANDING *YOUR* OCD: YOUR OWN VICIOUS FLOWER

We have discussed examples of the most common forms of OCD. However, for each person, even for each person with one of these types, the exact meaning and details of the particular processes that are keeping the OCD going will be different, personal and unique. Therefore it is important to use this chapter to think about the particular processes involved in your own OCD. See page 275 for a blank vicious flower diagram. Do not worry if you cannot yet fill in all of the boxes; this will be a work in progress.

Firstly, think of a recent time when you were particularly bothered by the problem. Getting a clear example will help you analyse what happens in your OCD. It's useful to think of a recent time, or an example which you can clearly remember. You are going to think back to that situation and go through it in some detail in order to get the information to complete your vicious flower. Go back in your mind to that day and really try to bring as much detail as you can about it to the front of your mind: Where were you? What day and what time was it? Who were you with? What was your frame of mind?

Once you have set the scene, try to pinpoint when the OCD began to bother you. This is usually when an obsession, that is, an intrusive thought, doubt, image or urge, popped into your mind. Think about the moment when the intrusive thought entered your mind. Ask yourself:

'When I had the thought [..........] what, at the time, seemed like the worst thing that could happen? If that really did happen, what would it mean about me?

*What did it seem that having the thought could mean about me?'*

You should now have an idea of the meaning of the thought for you at the time that it bothered you. We now need to look at how you reacted and responded when this meaning was activated. Firstly consider the emotional responses to that meaning. Ask yourself:

*'When I thought that having this intrusion meant that [.............] what did I feel?'*

You may have felt anxious, worried or afraid, or uncomfortable. Sometimes people feel other emotions such as depression, anger and disgust, to name a few. Write down all the feelings that apply.

The next category of things to think about is your behavioural responses, things you actively did to manage the discomfort or fear or simply to stop something bad from happening. Ask yourself *'What did I feel I needed to do?'* Make sure you include things you did physically (such as checking, washing, or doing a ritual), but also think about things you did mentally, inside your head (such as replacing bad thoughts with good ones, pushing the thoughts away, saying a prayer, arguing with the thought).

You now need to think about where your attention was at this moment. Ask yourself:

*'What did I pay attention to? Was I "looking for trouble?"'*

Finally, ask yourself:

*'Did I do anything else to try to deal with it?'*

If they apply, you may want to include slightly longer-term processes such as avoidance and getting reassurance from others in the diagram.

You should now have something that resembles a flower. Use the case examples to help you think about all of the behaviours and responses that keep your belief in danger going. Do not worry about differences or if you have more or fewer 'petals' to your vicious flower.

### Getting the vicious bit

So you have now thought through the intrusion and the meaning, and the different responses that resulted from that meaning being activated. The arrows out from the meaning represent the fact that the meaning causes these things to happen. However, as we have discussed in detail above, there is a two-way process going on, a vicious circle. Have a look at your responses in each petal of the flower and consider what effect this response has on the central meaning. Does it make it seem more or less believable? Be careful to distinguish between whether the responses help you feel better in the short term and whether in the long term they strengthen the belief in the meaning connected with the intrusive thought. If you are not sure, go back to the previous section on how OCD takes and keeps hold for information on specific processes.

It is worth having a go at a few different examples to see if it always works in the same way for you. If you experience several different forms of OCD, then it is worth drawing a vicious flower for each type. Think about how the processes are similar or different in each case. Think about whether the central meaning is similar or different.

# SUMMARY

OCD stays around because of a number of processes that keep a belief in danger going. The particular processes may be slightly different for each individual. You will see from reading this book that even though there are many types of OCD, the fundamentals of the way OCD works are the same in each case, even if the details differ. It is important to understand how OCD works across the range of types of OCD to see how it might work for you.

# 5
# STARTING TO TACKLE YOUR PROBLEM

The previous chapter should have helped you understand the detailed way you respond to your fear and they way in which this can keep the central meaning going and therefore lock the OCD in place. By now it should be clear that the basis of the anxiety and discomfort you experience as OCD is an effect of the entirely understandable way in which (1) you have come to see (misinterpret) your intrusive thoughts as more dangerous than they really are, and (2) these misinterpretations motivate and drive reactions which keep the sense of threat going, or even increase it. It is not possible, of course, simply to 'stop it'; if it were, you would have done it already. In this chapter we introduce the crucial idea of looking for an alternative way of thinking about the responsibility and threat meanings which sit at the heart of OCD, and help you think about how to consider the evidence and implications of such an alternative. Before we do that, we want to explain why developing and working on an alternative explanation can be so powerfully helpful. We will do that by using an example: think about the following situation.

*Imagine that you are sitting at the kitchen table one day, and hear a bleep. It is your partner/husband/wife's phone. You look at it and see it's a text from your best friend, arranging a meeting the next day. You see more texts of the same type and see there are lots of phone calls. You can't make sense of it, but are worried so you take a deep breath and ask your partner what this is about.*

*Several possibilities might happen.*

1. *Your partner offers you 'reassurance'. They say not to worry, there is nothing in it, forget about it. Often people with OCD are given this type of reassurance … they are told not to worry, there is no truth to their fears. Unfortunately this doesn't help. Why? Well, in order to feel better, the person needs to make sense of what is really going on. They need an alternative explanation.*

2. *Your partner smiles, and tells you that they and your best friend have been arranging a surprise birthday party for you. Obviously the surprise is now gone, which is a shame, but you are likely to stop feeling worried.*

The key to being able to tackle your OCD is having a sensible alternative explanation which allows you to understand the things you previously thought dangerous. That's what this book is about; making sense of your OCD in ways which allow you to see what's really going on, rather than being stuck in your fears about it.

By now you should have a good idea of the sorts of things that keep OCD going and we hope that you have been able to use this knowledge to gain some idea of what may be contributing to your own OCD problem hanging around. In this chapter we introduce the idea of an alternative to your meaning and will consider the evidence and implications of this alternative. We will use the examples from Chapter 4 to illustrate what needs to happen to break free from OCD. Using these examples, we will also guide you through understanding and tackling your own problem.

Throughout the last two chapters we have used the 'vicious flower' (what therapists often call formulation), which is our diagram that helps us to understand the counterproductive nature of safety-seeking behaviours and other ways of reacting to the responsibility meanings which go with OCD. The vicious flower is in fact a summary of the alternative explanation of how OCD works. This diagram helped us to see how OCD worked for Jennifer, Suse, Johnson and Jeremy.

# THEORY A/B

At the centre of the vicious flower is the key meaning that drives the problem for each person. For the people in our examples, and for you if you have OCD, that meaning has been treated as though it is a fact and life has been lived accordingly. But what if this key meaning is not a fact at all, but a belief that can be examined? What if this key meaning is not a helpful way, or even the 'right' way of thinking about the problem at all? OCD has convinced you for a long time that something bad may happen and that it is your responsibility to do something about it; this belief, in whatever form it exists for you, has fuelled all your safety-seeking behaviours and the other reactions involved in locking OCD in place. It is important to say that striving to keep yourself and others safe is both a logical and normal response if you believe that there is danger and that you can do something about it. However, we need to consider that there may be an altogether different way of thinking about the problem that you are experiencing. This is that, in fact, the problem is not one of danger at all, but one of *worry about danger.* Further than this, if the problem is worry about danger, then all of the very understandable measures you have been taking to avoid danger have in fact kept the problem of *worry* going and may even have made it much worse.

Take a minute to think about the difference between these two ways of thinking about what is going on and in particular think about what may fit best as a *description of your problem.* We call these two alternatives Theory A (the problem is danger) and Theory B (the problem is worry about danger). Some examples of these two ways of thinking about the problem are given below.

| THEORY A: OCD SAYS | THEORY B: OCD IS |
|---|---|
| My problem is that I might be careless and household appliances could catch fire and burn down the house | My problem is that I am a careful person who worries about household appliances catching fire and burning down the house |
| My problem is that I will get contaminated with dirt, disease and germs and die | My problem is that I am a clean person who worries a lot that I will get contaminated with dirt, disease and germs and die |
| My problem is that I am a wicked person because my thoughts are blasphemous and I will be condemned for them | My problem is that I am a person who is committed to my faith and because of this I worry my thoughts are blasphemous and I will be condemned for them |
| My problem is that I might be a child abuser who could harm a child | My problem is that I am a very caring person who worries that I might harm a child |

You may be looking at Theory A thinking that, well if that was true, of course I would worry about it! This is very logical, and it would mean that Theory A was a better explanation of what is happening than Theory B. Theory B is the idea that the problem *itself* is one of excessive worry. This is not to say that a Theory B is 'just' a worry problem and therefore not serious as everyone with OCD knows all too well! Worry problems are serious and significant. Consider these two alternatives as competing explanations for the problem, and think about which one makes the best sense of your experiences. In this sense they **cannot both be true**.

## EVIDENCE FOR THEORY A/B

Given that Theory A and B are very different ways of considering the problem, they will have very different implications as to what you do about it. Therefore it is important to think firstly about which of these two theories is the one that *best fits with your experience, both now and in the past*. The first step towards comparing them is to *examine the evidence* for each of the theories. When doing this, we need you to be as unbiased as possible, so look out for whether you are applying double standards, or accepting any ambiguous evidence. You can think about all the things which may support each theory – these could include things that have happened to you, things that have happened to others, as well as the opinions of others and how people generally behave. When we consider the evidence for each alternative, we need to act almost as though we are in a court, with the same high standards applied to our evidence. Is the evidence reliable or merely circumstantial? Are the character witnesses trustworthy?

## JENNIFER'S CHECKING OCD

We will use Jennifer's example (see page 88) for her checking problem first.

| THEORY A: OCD SAYS | THEORY B: OCD IS |
|---|---|
| The problem is that household appliances could catch fire if I am not careful enough | The problem is that I worry about household appliances catching fire |
| **Evidence:** | **Evidence:** |
| This happened in a student flat | I don't actually know what caused the fire I read about. I haven't actually heard of this happening to anyone so it must be very rare |

| **Evidence:** | **Evidence:** |
|---|---|
| *(This happened in a student flat)* | *I have often worried about things in the past but I could rely on others checking for me so it didn't become such a problem* |
| | *Nobody else is doing these checks. Perhaps I just worry more than others about it. Everyone else says I do!* |

The first piece of evidence that came to mind for Jennifer's Theory A was the newspaper story about a fire in a student flat that she had read around the time her problem began to get worse. When she thought more about this, she realised that this was an ambiguous piece of evidence, as she did not know the cause of the fire and had assumed that it was to do with an electrical fault. This may have been the cause of the fire, but she did not know for certain. When she thought about all the people she knew and all of the electrical appliances that they had, often switched on all of the time and certainly not checked or unplugged, it occurred to her that she had not heard of any fires being caused by them. Jennifer concluded that, although it could happen, it must be quite rare. This led her to think about Theory B, that perhaps her problem was excessive worrying about this event. She asked herself whether she was a worrier in general. She was certainly aware that other people thought she worried too much, and recognised that this had been part of her personality since childhood, which supported the idea that her experiences may be part of a worry problem.

## SUSE'S CONTAMINATION OCD

Look at the example below for the contamination problems that bothered Suse (see page 98):

| THEORY A: OCD SAYS | THEORY B: OCD IS |
|---|---|
| The problem is that I will get contaminated with dirt, germs or disease and die | The problem is that I worry that I will get contaminated with dirt, germs or disease and die |
| **Evidence:** | **Evidence:** |
| People die from MRSA in hospital | I have often worried about things in the past |
| | I have read lots of magazine articles about diseases that have made me worry more – it is actually very rare for people to catch these diseases and die |

When she thought about why Theory A seemed so convincing, Suse brought to mind several stories she had read about people dying in hospital from MRSA, and realised that she found this very frightening. She had never been ill or to hospital and was quite afraid of the idea. She noticed that she was a person who was very tuned in to issues of health and illness. When she considered Theory B, she realised that she had spent a lot of time focusing on her fears and that this had contributed to making her worry worse. She always noticed and, in fact, looked out for, the very rare cases of illness rather than thinking about the millions of people who are exposed to all sorts of germs all the time and do not die. She had not helped this bias by looking on the internet and reading sensationalist magazines.

## JEREMY'S RUMINATION OCD

Let's turn to Jeremy's problem of doubts that he might want to harm his or other children (see page 112).

| THEORY A: OCD SAYS | THEORY B: OCD IS |
|---|---|
| The problem is that I might harm a child | The problem is that I worry that I might harm a child |
| **Evidence:** | **Evidence:** |
| The thoughts make me feel very anxious | Feeling anxious is not evidence that I will act on the thoughts. The fact that the thoughts make me feel anxious means that I do not want to act on them |

Jeremy was very troubled by his thoughts that he might harm a child. When he began thinking about Theory A, he could not come up with any historical reasons or evidence that he was capable of harming anyone, let alone a child. However, the feelings of anxiety and dread were so strong when he experienced the thoughts, that he found it very hard to dismiss them completely. He was sure that they must mean something. The strong sensations of anxiety were almost overwhelming, to the extent that he feared he might somehow lose control and act on the thoughts.

## JOHNSON'S RELIGIOUS OCD

Let us consider Johnson's problem (see page 121) in the same way.

| **THEORY A: OCD SAYS** | **THEORY B: OCD IS** |
| --- | --- |
| The problem is that my thoughts are blasphemous and I will be condemned for them | The problem is that I worry my thoughts are blasphemous and I will be condemned for them |
| **Evidence:** | **Evidence:** |
| It is a sin to have sexual images when you are in church or thinking about God | The images are not things I want to think about and they make me feel very anxious |
| | I have always tried to live a very Christian life and there is no other evidence that I am a bad person |
| | I worry about this because I am religious |

Johnson first considered the evidence for Theory A. He had certainly been taught in church that some thoughts and actions were sinful and was worried that his thoughts would come into this category. However, when he thought about Theory B as an explanation for his experiences, he wondered whether the fact that he was so distressed by these thoughts said more about the nature of the problem. If he had not been disturbed by the thoughts, he would have been experiencing them in a different way, with enjoyment. When he thought about the images, he realised that they were always very upsetting when they came. Although he struggled to be clear about where the images came from and was worried that he might be being tempted by the devil, there was certainly no enjoyment of them when they did appear and he realised that he did not want to experience them. He had always tried to live according to the teachings of his faith and always considered his religion when making decisions in life.

## BE OBJECTIVE

When looking at evidence we need to be careful about emotions. We said earlier that it is likely that when you are carrying out your compulsions they generally *feel* necessary as they feel like they have helped you avert a danger, or helped your anxiety decrease a bit. However, if things *feel* necessary, that is not the same as meaning that they are necessary. Consider times when you are feeling less anxious, and if the drive to complete the compulsions is as strong.

---

**LOOK OUT FOR THE FOLLOWING OCD TRAPS WHEN CONSIDERING EVIDENCE FOR THEORY A/B**

- **Ambiguous or circumstantial evidence.** Just because two things happened at the same time, it does not mean that one caused the other.
- **Biases.** Are you just thinking about the one case where something went wrong and ignoring the many cases when it did not?
- **Double standards.** Are you applying much harsher rules for yourself than you would for other people? Or judging yourself from a point of view (now) of having more information than you did at the time.
- **Overvaluing your responsibility.** Is your sense of responsibility working overtime?
- **Feelings as evidence.** Are you taking anxiety itself as evidence that there is something to fear?

---

## IMPLICATIONS OF THEORY A/B – WHAT FOLLOWS FROM EACH

In all of the examples above, there is very little hard evidence on the side of Theory A at all, and in each case, Theory B seems to fit much better as an explanation of the person's problems. But let's not stop there. Remember that a version of Theory A is very likely to have been, up to now, how you have been defining your problem. There is more work to do in terms of considering what it really means to live according to either of these two theories. We need to know what follows from each theory, what each one means in terms of the principles you need to apply. The next thing to think about then is, if Theory A or Theory B was true, and you believed it wholeheartedly, what would that mean you needed to do? Let's take each one separately. Remember to treat each theory as a definite statement of the problem, so don't hold back! We are working out what would need to happen if the problem was *definitely* one of danger or *definitely* one of worry.

### Implications for Jennifer's checking OCD

Jennifer considered her checking problem using the boxes below. Firstly she considered Theory A.

---

**THEORY A: OCD SAYS**

The problem is that household appliances could catch fire

**What do I need to do?**

Check all the appliances to make sure they are safe

Try to remember how I checked as I do it

Get other people to check as well

Get rid of household appliances/ never go out

**THEORY B: OCD IS**

The problem is that I worry about household appliances catching fire.

**What do I need to do?**

---

When Jennifer began to consider the behaviours that followed from taking Theory A as 100% true, she wrote down a list of rules which were in fact almost exactly what she had been doing. She had been checking and taking a lot of precautions. However, even though she felt compelled to do these things, there had been some doubt in her mind about whether these precautions were excessive. She was certainly aware that most people did not take the same measures that she did and although her belief that the problem of danger was high, and very high when she was anxious, it was not 100%. When she thought about it, she realised that what logically followed from Theory A was that her checks might not be adequate. Really, she should encourage other people to do the checks as well. But of course other people could make a mistake as much as she could, and so the safest thing was never to go out at all. *Taken to its logical conclusion*, total faith in Theory A meant that she should restrict all of her activities and those of other people. Jennifer had restricted her life to such a degree that she could see how far she had gone towards this. At this point, we also wanted Jennifer to consider what will happen if she continues to follow the rules of Theory A even as much as she has been doing.

| THEORY A: OCD SAYS | THEORY B: OCD IS |
|---|---|
| *The problem is that household appliances could catch fire* | *The problem is that I worry about household appliances catching fire* |
| **If I keep following these rules, what will happen in the future?** | **If I keep following these rules, what will happen in the future?** |
| *I will need to do more and more checking; this will take over my life. I will have no life* | |

| If I keep following these rules, what will happen in the future? | If I keep following these rules, what will happen in the future? |
| --- | --- |
| *I will be an anxious mess because I can never be completely certain I have eliminated all the danger* | |

For Jennifer, continuing to follow the rules of Theory A would mean that her life would have been subsumed into constant checking. She would never go out again. The thought of this made Jennifer feel very sad and anxious. However, this is what *could* happen if Jennifer continued along this pathway. She then began to consider Theory B, and the implications if this was definitely true as a description of the problem.

What struck her first was that, if Theory B was true, then she did not need to do any checks, or any more than the 'average' person. She realised that, if the problem was worry, then the way to deal with that was to not give in to the worry. The checks had been increasing her preoccupation with danger and had undermined her trust in herself. Therefore she needed to build this up again by testing out her fears and facing up to the worry. If Theory B was true, and she treated the problem as though it was one of worry, then doing these things should help her overcome that problem.

| THEORY A: OCD SAYS | THEORY B: OCD IS |
| --- | --- |
| *The problem is that household appliances could catch fire* | *The problem is that I worry about household appliances catching fire* |

### What do I need to do?

Check all the appliances to make sure they are safe

Try to remember how I checked

Get other people to check as well

Get rid of household appliances/ never go out

### If I keep following these rules, what will happen in the future?

I will need to do more and more checking; this will take over my life. I will have no life

I will be an anxious mess because I can never be completely certain I have eliminated all the danger

### What do I need to do?

Don't check ... more than once. Aim to not check at all!

Face up to the worry

Challenge the thoughts

### If I keep following these rules, what will happen in the future?

I should become less anxious

I can go out again and be normal

---

## Implications for Suse's contamination OCD

Next, Suse examined her problems using the same methods. Firstly she thought about the rules that followed from belief in Theory A. As Jennifer had discovered, what she had been doing corresponded with Theory A, but when she questioned herself as to whether the rules were enough, the logical conclusion of Theory A was to go even further, wash more, avoid more and get other people to do the same. A future lived according to these rules would be like a prison camp. Suse realised that it would take up more and more of her time to follow the rules and that she would have to increasingly restrict her life. When she thought about Theory B, it was clear that she would not need to wash excessively. It occurred to her that it might be better not to wash at all, to test out her worries. She certainly did not need to act every time she had a thought that something could be contaminated. After all, she was bound to have lots of those thoughts if she was worried about it! A future lived according to these principles was one of freedom and much less anxiety.

| **THEORY A: OCD SAYS** | **THEORY B: OCD IS** |
|---|---|
| The problem is that I will get contaminated with dirt, germs or disease and die | The problem is that I worry that I will get contaminated with dirt, germs or disease and die |
| **If this is true, what do I need to do?** | **If this is true, what do I need to do?** |
| Wash my hands at least 50 times a day; use alcohol gel and wet wipes | Ignore thoughts about disease |
| Wash hands until they 'feel right' | Treat worries as worries – not as signs of imminent danger |
| Use anti-bacterial spray several times a day on all surfaces | Freely touch things when out in public without washing my hands |
| Keep on the lookout for brown or red marks on objects | |
| Ensure that I don't spread germs or disease to others | |
| **If I keep following these rules, what will happen in the future?** | **If I keep following these rules, what will happen in the future?** |
| I will need to do more and more cleaning and checking; this will take over my life | I can do what I like with my life |

A further question that Suse considered was what it might mean about her as a person if each theory was true.

---

**What does this say about me as a person?**

*I'm vulnerable*

**What does this say about me as a person?**

*I am sensitive and I have a worry or anxiety problem but I am no more vulnerable than anyone else*

*I am a determined person who wants to tackle this problem*

---

## Implications for Jeremy's rumination OCD

Jeremy started to think about what it really meant to live according to the rules his fear dictated. He was already spending hours a day trying to work out what the thoughts meant but when he considered it, he realised that there was no end to that as he would never feel safe or sure enough. It made him feel very sad to think that it meant he would not really be able to be around his daughter. When he came to think about Theory B it was hard to see the problem being worry as a real alternative, as he was so used to thinking about the problem as one of potential danger. However, if he 'tried on' Theory B for size and thought about what it would mean if it were true, he came up with a set of principles that were in essence the opposite of what he was doing. If the problem really was worry, then worrying about it could obviously only make it worse, like digging to get out of a hole! What he needed to do was to *stop* taking his thoughts so seriously and stop trying to work them out. It would also mean that he was safe to do whatever was required and if he continued to do that he would have more time for his wife and baby and be a better father and husband.

| THEORY A: OCD SAYS | THEORY B: OCD IS |
|---|---|
| The problem is that I might harm a child | The problem is that I worry that I might harm a child |
| **If this is true, what do I need to do?** | **If this is true, what do I need to do?** |
| Monitor myself for signs of going mad or moral slipping | Ignore thoughts |
| Avoid coffee or alcohol, to stay in control | Treat worries as worries — not as signs of imminent danger |
| Get my wife to look after the baby. Avoid all children | Spend more time with the baby, even after drinking coffee |
|  | Stop questioning myself |
| **If I keep following these rules, what will happen in the future?** | **If I keep following these rules, what will happen in the future?** |
| I will never be safe enough | I will get to spend time with my baby and wife and enjoy being a (good) dad and uncle, etc. |
| I will feel very sad — my daughter will not know me |  |

Jeremy thought about what Theory A and B said about him as a person. When he reflected on this, one thing was completely clear to him in all the muddle of his thoughts: he truly wanted to be a good person and play a full role in his family. It made sense that all his rumination and avoidance was designed to *protect others* which only a caring and sensitive person would do. It was also what others had said about him on many occasions, despite his own fears.

| **What does this say about me as a person?** | **What does this say about me as a person?** |
|---|---|
| *I'm bad and dangerous* | *I'm sensitive and caring* |

*Implications for Johnson's religious OCD*

Johnson thought about his problem with having unwanted thoughts about his religion. He wrote down his Theory A, what he felt he needed to do when he was upset and anxious, when OCD was telling him that he was a blasphemer who would be condemned. He realised that trying to avoid having the thoughts had been very unhelpful, and would mean that in the future he would have to avoid everything about his religion. This made him feel very sad. When he thought about his Theory B, as a problem of anxiety and worry, he understood that he did not need to try to avoid triggers or the thoughts themselves, as the intrusive thoughts were just thoughts. He realised it was counterproductive to monitor his thoughts and his body as this made him more anxious and more likely to experience intrusive thoughts. Johnson felt optimistic when he considered what life would be like for him in the future when he lived his life with Theory B – he would be free to enjoy his faith in a way consistent with how he really was as a person.

| **THEORY A: OCD SAYS** | **THEORY B: OCD IS** |
|---|---|
| *The problem is that my thoughts are blasphemous and I will be condemned for them* | *The problem is that I worry that my thoughts are blasphemous and I will be condemned for them* |

**If this is true, what do I need to do?**

*Try to push the thoughts out of my mind*

*Look out for the thoughts*

*Try to atone for them at every opportunity*

*Avoid situations where the thoughts could be triggered*

*Stay away from church*

**If I keep following these rules, what will happen in the future?**

*I will need to do more praying and avoiding; this will take over my life*

**What does this say about me as a person?**

*I'm a bad person*

**If this is true, what do I need to do?**

*Ignore the thoughts*

*Not monitor my thoughts or my body*

*Go to church and study the Bible regardless of any intrusive thoughts*

*Not avoid anywhere or anything*

**If I keep following these rules, what will happen in the future?**

*I will have a closer relationship with God and my church*

**What does this say about me as a person?**

*I am a good and religious person, who takes their religion and morals very seriously*

# THEORY A AND B – SO HOW DO I KNOW WHICH IS RIGHT?

While it is important to think about the two theories and which applies best, we don't want to spend a great deal of time trying to 'disprove' Theory A – imagine if Suse (contamination fears) got tempted into this kind of thinking:

*'Perhaps I am too anxious about dirt and germs. I'll go and look up on the internet how likely it really is that I will die from salmonella, and I'll investigate how long it stays "live" on your hands so I know when it is safe to touch other things. I'll ask everyone I know how often they wash their hands; once I know this I'll wash my hands a bit more than them, to be on the safe side.'*

Can you see what the problem might be with this? Once Suse starts looking on the internet she will find all sorts of information that will furnish her with various contradictory 'facts' that may increase her uncertainty, or set up a new set of obsessional rules that might be quicker but would still be generated from a belief about being responsible for preventing harm. Asking everyone she knows how often they wash their hands could end up being a form of reassurance if she has in mind that there is a 'right answer'.

It can be useful to ask other people about their behaviour, for example, how often they wash their hands, if you have lost track of what is 'normal' or typical. What you are likely to find is a huge range of behaviour. Some people do wash their hands frequently; other people might only do so a few times a day. The important information to gain from a 'survey' of other people's behaviour is to establish a flexible approach. The goal is *to be able to* not wash your hands even if you prefer to at other times. For example, if you are at home, you may prefer to wash your hands before preparing food. However, if you are out camping or having a picnic, this might not be possible – the goal is *to be able to* get on with eating in these circumstances and to *take the risk* that you might pick up a bug. Remember the insurance metaphor we described in Chapter 4 – you may feel like the compulsions are protecting you from something terrible happening. This is a very nice idea, but the cost of carrying them out 'effectively' enough is very high. It's a bit like buying a house insurance policy that protects against everything but costs £1 million per year. So the question is, how much are you really paying to carry out your OCD compulsions?

Often, obsessional concerns include negative consequences in the longer term, i.e. not doing your rituals today could lead to a family member having an accident at any point in the future. This is when it is useful to build up evidence for Theory B. We can never be sure that nothing bad will ever happen; what we do know is that making a constant effort to prevent something bad happening inevitably increases your preoccupation with and belief in Theory A.

This also shows something else important ... that it is possible to care too much. We have noticed over the years that most people with OCD care too much for their own good, but are reluctant to give this up in case it results in them being responsible for harm to themselves or other people. Fortunately, it is possible to change this and escape from the trap which is OCD while still being a caring person.

The more you go about your life acting as if Theory B is true, the more you will find out how the world really works without OCD. OCD (Theory A) has been telling you for a long time that terrible things will happen. What we know is that Theory B predicts that when you stop doing safety-seeking behaviour, and stop avoiding anything, your thoughts will become less troubling, your feelings of anxiety will subside and you will start to enjoy life a great deal more.

---

**KEY IDEA**

OCD *says* the problem is danger and you must spend all your time preventing it. OCD *is* a problem of worry about danger.

---

Try to fill in a Theory A and Theory B for your problems in the table on page 276.

## REVISIT YOUR GOALS

Are there any Theory A ideas in your goals? Watch out for goals that are actually ways of doing your rituals more quickly, or that are forms of avoidance. You may have a goal like 'stop having intrusive thoughts', which would be counterproductive.

Following working on Theory A/B, here are some of the goals of Jennifer, Suse, Jeremy and Johnson:

## JENNIFER (CHECKING OCD)
*Short term:*
- Get to my classes on time
- Go out with my flat mates

*Medium term:*
- Invite people over to flat

*Long term:*
- Live alone

## SUSE (CONTAMINATION OCD)
*Short term:*
- Only wash my hands after using the toilet
- Go on the bus

*Medium term:*
- Cook dinner for a friend

*Long term:*
- Go on a long holiday abroad

## JEREMY (RUMINATION OCD)
*Short term:*
- Change my daughter's nappy
- Spend time on my own with my daughter

*Medium term:*
- Babysit for other children

*Long term:*
- Have another baby

## JOHNSON (RELIGIOUS OCD)
*Short term:*
- Go to church
- Meet up with friends

*Medium term:*
- Go on a church outing for the day

*Long term:*
- Train as a lay preacher

# CHALLENGING YOUR OCD

We talked above about the fact that people who suffer from anxiety do so because they think things are more dangerous than they really are. If you think about the potential dangers of any situation then it is all too easy to see really dangerous possibilities, and having seen these, it can be fiendishly difficult to ignore them. It is really hard to think your way out of anxiety without checking it out in the real world, and in the end that's what you have to do. So, if Theory B is correct, then these situations which have dominated your life are not as dangerous as you thought. How to check it out? In the first instance, it's best to gather information about whether Theory B is correct. For most people suffering from OCD, this is a very new way of thinking and working, but extremely useful when you get going. The best way to get going on it is to test it out. That's what a lot of the behavioural experiments described next are about. Once you feel a lot more confident from this that Theory B might be right, that your problem may be one of being worried about danger rather than being *in* danger, you will need to take a deep breath and do some behavioural experiments to test out which is best. That's what this next section is about.

## 'TAKING THE RISK'

Now you have a good understanding of how the problem works, hopefully it is clear what you need to do to get rid of OCD:

➤ **Start living your life according to Theory B**
➤ **Challenge your belief that you are responsible for preventing something bad happening (challenge Theory A)**
➤ **Don't avoid anything**
➤ **Stop all safety-seeking behaviours**
➤ **Start finding out how the world really works**

It is likely that at the moment the idea of doing this is still very anxiety-provoking – you might be thinking 'but what if something bad does happen?' or 'bad things do happen, why would I take the risk?' An important step to take in treatment is to acknowledge that *a bad thing has already happened – OCD has disrupted or even ruined months, years or decades of your life.* Standing up to OCD involves taking the risk that you will feel anxious, and taking the risk that something bad might happen. It takes courage to not wash your hands if you have been convinced for a long time that if you don't, you will die. It takes courage to not do your rituals if you have truly believed for a long time that those rituals keep people safe. When you *do* do things differently, you will find out that the OCD has been lying to you and bullying you all along.

## OCD BULLY

It can be useful to think of OCD as a bully. Think about the way a school bully goes about intimidating their victims. The bully approaches and demands 50p. The scared schoolchild hands over the money under the threat of violence. The next day the bully asks for £1. The next week £2. The schoolchild has to resort to taking money from their mother's purse to pay the bully. The threat of violence is too frightening so they keep paying.

One day the schoolchild decides they have had enough of being bullied and stands up the bully, refusing to hand over their money. The bully is not used to being challenged and turns out to be 'all mouth and no trousers' – he walks away sheepishly rather than have to carry out his threats. The bullied schoolchild feels proud that they overcame their fear and enjoys spending their money on what they want and walking around without feeling pre-occupied and scared.

OCD is like a bully, as the threat of something bad happening is frightening enough to keep 'paying the price' What OCD extorts from you grows over time – once you have started washing your hands three times, the OCD can easily bully you into washing them five times, or ten …

Standing up to the bully is frightening at first but OCD is like most bullies – the threats are just threats and if you stand up to them, they don't know what to do. Just imagine the satisfaction, relief and pleasure you will get from standing up to this problem.

# FINDING OUT HOW THE WORLD REALLY WORKS: BEHAVIOURAL EXPERIMENTS

Because Theory A and Theory B have such different implications for now and the future, it is extremely important to find out for yourself which one is true. The exciting thing is that this can be tested in the real world. In Cognitive Behaviour Therapy, we use the term 'behavioural experiment' to describe what we do to test out beliefs about the world. As the phrase suggests, a behavioural experiment is a planned test of a belief involving doing something differently from how you would usually do it, recording the results and using this new information to decide which theory fits best.

When you are tackling your problem, behavioural experiments will:

➤ Help you find out that the things that you fear do not happen
➤ Reveal the importance of your counterproductive safety-seeking behaviours in maintaining your anxiety and your belief that you are responsible for preventing harm
➤ Help you find out for yourself whether the alternative Theory B is more useful
➤ Enable you to discover how the world really works

## HOW MANY EXPERIMENTS DO I NEED TO DO?

The point of a behavioural experiment is to find out in a structured way what happens if you go against the OCD. It is good to try things a couple of times to see if you get the same results and if your anxiety lessens as we would predict. If it does, then you already have good information that the problem is worry and you need to incorporate this into your everyday life. Remember this is about how the world *really* works so it means that you can live your life without OCD.

# THE THREE CHOICES

Standing up to OCD can be very hard – if it was easy you would have got rid of this problem a long time ago. However, now you have got a good understanding of how OCD works and an idea of how to tackle it, let's think about how to make your fight against the problem as effective as possible.

## SPECIAL FORCES TRAINING

How would you train soldiers in the special forces? They need to be on top form to deal with extremely challenging situations at a moment's notice. Would you send them to a nice beach and instruct them to lounge about with a cocktail or two? Or would you insist on plenty of practice of dealing with difficult situations, with repeated exercises of what they would need to do? Assuming you chose the second option, of repeated practice and training – why was that? It makes sense to practise so that next time the soldiers are called into action they are well prepared mentally and physically for what confronts them.

Dealing with your OCD problem is similar – you need to practise dealing with the difficult situations that catch you out. If you really go for it with your behavioural experiments, the next time an intrusive thought pops into your head and your OCD beliefs and anxiety kick in, you will be prepared and know what to do. In treatment we encourage taking the fight to the OCD bully by being 'anti-obsessional'.

When you are planning your behavioural experiments to get rid of your problem, keep these 'three choices' in mind:

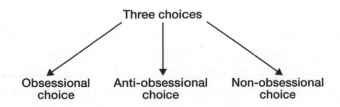

1. *The obsessional choice* – this is the one you do already when OCD convinces you that you need to do something to stop something bad happening. (For Jennifer this is checking appliances, for Suse, washing her hands, for Johnson avoiding his Bible study, for Jeremy saying 'I don't want you to die, I'll keep you safe'.)

2. *The non-obsessional choice* – this is what Theory B suggests you should be doing to be free of the problem (not checking, no hand-washing, no avoiding, no repeating 'neutralising' phrases).

3. *The anti-obsessional choice* – this is what you need to do to stand up to the problem. In effect, this means doing the opposite of what OCD wants you to do, or by going much further than the non-obsessional choice to see what happens.

---

**THE BUILDER'S APPRENTICE**

When a young lad started on a building site, the men on the site played a well-known trick on him, asking the poor boy to hold up a (solid) wall that they had just built. Of course the apprentice did what he was told and he believed that if he let go of the wall then it would fall down, with serious consequences for the wall and for him. This was such a terrible thing for him to imagine that he stood 'holding the wall up' for hours. In fact, the joke went so well that the rest of the labourers actually left and went home.

What could he have done to find out if they were playing a trick on him? The obvious thing to do would have been to let go, to find out what would happen, that what he believed was not true. However, if he just let go, and found out that the wall stood, he might still think that the wall was not very stable. The best way he could have tested things out and gone home with confidence would have been if he

> not only let go, but pushed the wall hard. In this way, he would have found out that it was completely solid. This is the equivalent of doing things the anti-obsessional way.

We will look at specific examples of these choices in the following chapter.

## 'LETTING THOUGHTS GO'

Intrusive thoughts will continue to bother you as you are tackling this problem. You will need to practise 'letting the thoughts go' – they are insignificant and irrelevant, and do not need to be confronted, argued with, cancelled out or neutralised in any way. Any of those responses to the thoughts has the paradoxical effect of making the thoughts more salient and frequent. A useful metaphor is the 'unwelcome guest at a party': imagine you are at an enjoyable party, drinking your drink and enjoying conversation. Someone you really dislike comes through the door. You could run up to them and try to push them out the door, shouting and screaming at them and trying to get other people to help you. This will ruin the evening for you and many other people. This is like trying to 'do something' with your thoughts. Or, after you noticed their arrival, you could ignore the unwelcome guest. Even if they brush past you or remain in your sight for a while, carry on drinking your drink and enjoying your conversation. This is like ignoring your intrusive thoughts, even if they are rattling around in your thinking for a while.

## TOLERATING (SOME) UNCERTAINTY

The idea of 'tolerating uncertainty' is an important part of tackling an OCD problem. As we have discussed in earlier chapters, OCD can feel like being plagued with doubts and uncertainties. For some people this can be doubt about whether they shut the front door, for others about whether they have picked up a disease.

In behavioural experiments it is often important to 'tolerate' doubt and uncertainty. What we mean by this is to put up with it. Uncertainty is a part of life – we all live with the uncertainty of death, illness or what will happen tomorrow. We have all learned or become accustomed to living with this uncertainty. If we are not certain, that doesn't mean that we are completely uncertain. OCD may have convinced you that you need to be 100% certain about something – this is usually impossible anyway. In behavioural experiments, when you are doing things very differently from your obsessional ways, you will need to practise putting up with a difficult sense of uncertainty. As we will go on to examine, you might predict that you won't be able to cope with this, or that it will last for a long time – these are all ideas that can be tested out in behavioural experiments.

## Tolerating (some) anxiety

Challenging your problem does involve putting up with some anxiety. This sounds off-putting, but remember how much anxiety you experience every day due to OCD. Anxiety works in the same way in OCD as it does for any other fear or phobia. For example, if you were afraid of spiders and saw one in the garden, your anxiety would go right up and if you ran away it would go down again very quickly. However, you would remain afraid of spiders and would be as frightened the next time you saw one. In the same way, if you have an intrusive thought, you will feel a spike in anxiety. If you then do a ritual, leave the situation or do any other kind of safety-seeking behaviour, your anxiety temporarily goes down. However, as you have not changed your belief about your thoughts, your anxiety will jump up again at the next thought. Your belief that the thought meant danger and you needed to act on it is still there as you have no other information.

Behavioural treatments for OCD (sometimes called 'exposure and response prevention', ERP) work on the principle that everyone is capable of 'habituation' to anxiety – getting used to the anxiety over time. In ERP treatment you would be encouraged to do something such as touch a 'contaminated' object for ten minutes without washing your hands or taking any other measures. During those ten minutes your anxiety will go down; each time you attempt it your anxiety will be slightly less and will go down (provided you do no compulsions). Over time your overall anxiety will be greatly diminished.

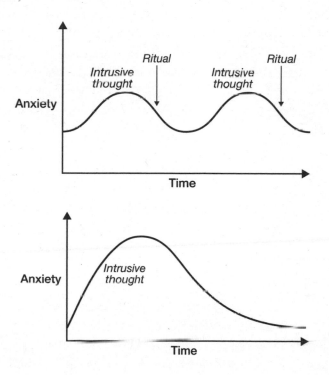

In CBT we have built on this principle when we use behavioural experiments. In each experiment we can predict that your anxiety will go up, and we make a prediction about how bad it will be and for how long. Then we can record whether it was as bad as you predicted. Most of the time behavioural experiments are designed to test out other ideas as well, such as whether someone actually becomes ill from contamination if you don't wash your hands, and to find out what happens to your beliefs about responsibility when you try to do things differently.

# DEALING WITH RESPONSIBILITY BELIEFS

As you will know from reading the previous chapters, having broad shoulders with regard to responsibility plays a very important role in the development of OCD, and in keeping it going. Because of an 'inflated sense of responsibility', people are motivated to try to stop bad things happening and become obsessional in their efforts to be safe enough. Therefore it goes without saying that in tackling the OCD and not doing what it is 'telling' you to do, you will feel *less* responsible and perhaps even irresponsible. This has probably been a very powerful reason to keep on doing compulsions and safety-seeking behaviours.

## CHALLENGING ALL-OR-NOTHING THINKING

Let's consider this idea a bit further and draw out a continuum of responsibility, with total responsibility on one end and total irresponsibility on the other end.

---

**CASE EXAMPLE**

*Mark lived with his parents; he spent hours each day straightening and ordering things round the house. He was really concerned that if he didn't have everything that he owned ordered and arranged in a particular, careful way something bad would happen to one of his parents. Some of his concern was about tangible risk, such as them falling down the stairs; some of his concern was about things not 'feeling right' – if things were not 'just so' that something bad would happen. He felt very strongly that he was responsible for their safety and that if anything bad happened to them it would be his fault, and that would make him a terrible, bad person.*

---

It is useful for Mark to draw up two continua:

1.  0% responsible – 100% responsible
2.  0% good – 100% good

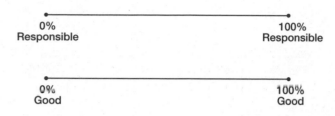

Mark thought that a person who gets very very drunk and drives home fast during the rush hour near to a school was 0% responsible and the controller of a nuclear power station was a good example of a 100% responsible person.

When Mark considered who he thought was at the end of a good–bad continuum, he thought that Hitler was 0% good and Mother Teresa was close to 100% good.

Mark undertook to disarrange his possessions and let his parents wander around freely. He was frightened that by changing his behaviour in this way this would be totally irresponsible and bad because he would be moving down the scale from Mother Teresa towards Hitler. The problem is that there are only two options there. Mark thought about some people that he knew and other famous people and placed them on this line. He found that these people generally fell somewhere between the two extremes – that is, few people are 100% good or bad, responsible or irresponsible. He was able to conclude that being more carefree around his house did not mean that he was irresponsible or bad and realised that OCD had tricked him into thinking in an 'all or nothing' way.

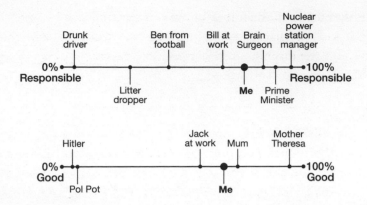

If you have OCD and spend much of your time thinking about the consequences of your actions and trying to stop bad things from happening, it is likely that you are nearer Mother Teresa and the controller of the nuclear power station than Hitler and the drunk driver.

On the responsibility continuum, think about where the *average* person is, which is likely to be somewhere near the middle. If you think about the average person (without OCD), who does not take *extra* precautions or worry *excessively* about their thoughts and actions, they are a long way from being totally irresponsible, and yet they are generally concerned and cautious when they need to be. If you have OCD, you will probably be much more 'responsible' than the average person, so changing and tackling your OCD will take you towards the normal and healthy middle range, where most people are.

You can also apply this continuum technique to ideas about cleanliness, perfectionism or anything else where you spot an 'all or nothing' bit of thinking. One of the tricks OCD uses is to get you to treat things as though they are black and white. Going through this exercise can help you see that for most things this is not true.

## CHALLENGING INFLATED RESPONSIBILITY

Because they are sensitive to ideas of responsibility, people with OCD can sometimes feel that things in the past were their fault, or that things in the future would be their fault to a huge degree. It's possible that if you think this, you may be seeing things through the magnification of inflated responsibility. Here are some examples:

---

**CASE EXAMPLE**

*Barbara once had a serious accident when driving a car and the other driver was badly injured. It had been wet weather and the other driver was driving fast and didn't look when coming into her lane. However, as she was unhurt in the accident, Barbara always worried that she was somehow responsible.*

---

Contributing factors and how much they influenced the accident:

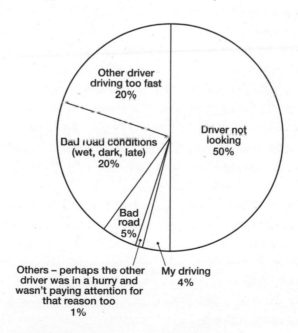

1. The other driver driving too fast = 20%
2. The driver not looking = 50%

3. Bad road conditions (wet, dark, late) = 20%
4. Bad road = 5%
5. Others – perhaps the other driver was in a hurry and wasn't paying attention for that reason too = 1%
6. My driving = 4%

Barbara concluded that her driving was a very small slice of the pie – this tiny sliver of influence was not the same as full responsibility. If the other 96% of the pie had not been there, there probably would not have been an accident.

---

**CASE EXAMPLE**
*When Charlie was younger he had a pet rabbit called Twiglet. He always said goodbye to Twiglet and gave him a stroke before he went off to school. One day he rushed off to school without stroking the rabbit and had the thought 'I hope Twiglet is okay' but when he returned the rabbit was not there and his parents had taken him to the vet to be put down. Charlie had not known that Twiglet was ill and always worried that because he had not said goodbye that he had somehow caused Twiglet's death. Because of this experience, over time Charlie developed the belief that his thoughts were important and he said rituals every night to keep those he loved 'safe' from harm. Even though he knew that these were pointless and couldn't really keep anyone safe, he felt very bad if he did not do the ritual, or did not do it properly due to his sense of responsibility.*

---

He thought about his earlier experience and the other factors that played a role in Twiglet's death:

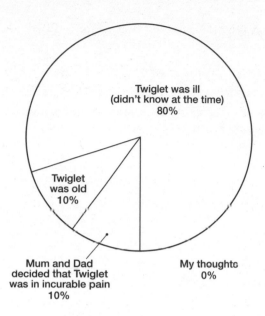

1. Twiglet was ill (didn't know at the time) = 80%
2. Twiglet was old = 10%
3. Mum and Dad decided that Twiglet was in incurable pain = 10%
4. My thoughts = 0%

Charlie knew on one level that it was unlikely his thoughts had 'caused' the death of his rabbit, but he had never really taken the time to consider the other factors that might have played a part. This was partly because this had happened when he was a child and he did not have the capacity to think things through in the same way as he did now. The original association he made was due to a coincidence, but his interpretation of this at the time had a lasting effect on his behaviour.

It is not necessary to completely change your views of responsibility in order to overcome OCD and there is nothing wrong with being a responsible person. However it is important to truly understand the role that *inflated* responsibility plays in keeping OCD going and how OCD might use that to stay around.

## SUMMARY

This chapter has explored an alternative way of thinking about your problem, that it is one of excessive worry rather than danger. Testing this out, accumulating evidence and acting accordingly is likely to help in your fight against OCD.

Purley Library

**Customer ID:** \*\*\*\*\*\*\*\*\*\*4713

**Items that you have borrowed**

Title: Break free from OCD
ID:    38015024129557
**Due: 01 August 2023**


Total items: 1
Account balance: £0.00
Borrowed: 1
Overdue: 0
Hold requests: 0
Ready for collection: 0
20/06/2023 17:22

Tel: 020 7884 5160
https://www.croydon.gov.uk/libraries-leisure-nd-culture/libraries

# 6
# BREAKING FREE FROM OCD

This chapter continues our case studies of the most common forms of OCD and guides you through specific examples of how to break free from those problems. It builds on what you have learnt in the last chapter about defining the problem in a completely different way and will show you in detail how seeing and treating OCD for what it is will help you move forward. We also discuss some of the common difficulties encountered in doing this and how you can overcome them.

## LETTING THOUGHTS GO

For most forms of OCD, the idea of 'letting thoughts go' is a useful one. As we have discussed in earlier chapters, in OCD it is not the thoughts themselves that are the problem. When breaking free from OCD, treat 'thoughts as thoughts' – not as danger signals, premonitions or signs that you are a bad person. In our examples below we will demonstrate how important it is to ignore or disregard the thoughts when you are challenging the problem. Remember the unwelcome guest at the party (page 161).

When you have a nagging doubt, such as 'Did I leave the door open' – it can be useful to think 'Maybe I did, maybe I didn't'. By doing this you are disengaging from the obsessional thought. Watch out for getting into a mental argument or for reassuring yourself, i.e. 'I did lock the door, it's fine' – this might make you feel less anxious for a short while, but as you know, you will only have to reassure or argue with yourself more.

# BREAKING FREE FROM CHECKING

In the previous chapters, we looked in detail at the processes and reactions that keep a checking problem going. We considered the problem as one of many vicious circles operating at the same time which fuel a sense of danger (Theory A). We have been looking at the example of Jennifer, who began to engage in a number of behaviours that fuelled her central belief that she was a potential danger. The more that she 'bought in' to this idea and acted accordingly, the worse and more severe her checking problem (and belief in Theory A) became. Although not clear to her when she was in the grip of her OCD, what she was doing was like trying to put out a fire by throwing petrol on it. It was suggested to Jennifer that there was an alternative way of thinking about her problem, that her *real* problem was one of extreme anxiety about danger (Theory B) and that her measures to try to manage danger had actually served to make her anxiety worse. Her Theory A/B table is below:

| THEORY A: OCD SAYS | THEORY B: OCD IS |
|---|---|
| The problem is that household appliances could catch fire and burn down the house | A problem of worry about household appliances catching fire and burning down the house |
| **Evidence:** | **Evidence:** |
| This happened in a student flat | I don't actually know what caused the fire I read about. I haven't heard of this happening to anyone so it must be very rare |

**Evidence:**

This happened in a student flat

**Evidence:**

I have often worried about things in the past but I could rely on others checking for me so it didn't become such a problem

Nobody else is doing these checks. Perhaps I just worry more than others about it. Everyone else says I do!

**If this is true, what do I need to do?**

Check all the appliances to make sure they are safe

Try to remember how I checked

Get other people to check as well

Get rid of household appliances/ never go out

**If this is true, what do I need to do?**

Don't check ... more than once

Face up to the worry

Challenge the thoughts

**What does this say about the future?**

I will need to do more and more checking; this will take over my life. I will have no life

I will be an anxious mess because I can never be completely certain I have eliminated all the danger

**What does this say about the future?**

I should become less anxious

I can go out again and be normal

| What does this say about me as a person? | What does this say about me as a person? |
|---|---|
| *Careless* | *Careful and caring person* |

Jennifer was excited by the possibility that there was another way of thinking and going about things that was very different to the OCD way she was so familiar with. A large part of her could see how compelling the case was for Theory B, particularly when she had to consider the evidence for both and could not really come up with much for Theory A. However, like most people with OCD, Jennifer was a very logical and intelligent person. She already knew that her problem was 'excessive' but felt so locked into the behaviours that it was very difficult to just stop them, particularly when she felt very anxious, which was much of the time. If you have a checking problem, understanding the problem provides an important basis to doing things differently. It may not be a case of just stopping, but testing out whether Theory B is a better fit for the difficulties you are experiencing and building up evidence for Theory B by testing things out. As described on page 156, it is much easier to give up a threatening idea when we have begun to see how the alternative way of thinking would work. Even better if we have also begun to gather evidence for the less threatening alternative.

In treatment we do ask people to stop checking and undertake behavioural experiments to find out what happens when they don't check. It's more than simply riding out your anxiety in the feared situation: you will also be testing out particular beliefs that you are responsible for harm by seeing what happens when you don't check. We always acknowledge that there is a risk that something bad will happen if you don't check, but the guarantee with continued checking is that OCD will always remain a problem.

## WHERE TO START?

People with checking OCD will often say, 'It's normal to check a bit, so where do I start?' It is a good idea to start with not checking at all in order to find out what happens. After this you can continue doing things in an anti-obsessional way to build up as much evidence as possible as to what happens when you don't do what OCD tells you. You can decide what rules you would like to live your life by once the OCD has gone. Remember that because of the way OCD works, it plays on a very broad sense of responsibility to drive the problem, so it is likely that you will feel uncomfortable when you start to do things differently. You may think of many catastrophes and how it is your job to prevent them. However, what you may not know is if you don't act in an obsessional way, *what happens next*. When you set up your own behavioural experiments, think about what the OCD is telling you will happen if you don't do what it says (write down your specific predictions and how much you believe them). Include in this column your prediction about how intense the anxiety will get (0–100%) and how long the anxiety will last.

## JENNIFER'S BEHAVIOURAL EXPERIMENT

**COMPLETE BEFORE THE EXPERIMENT**

| Planned behavioural experiment | Specific predictions and how much I believe them |
| --- | --- |
| Leave house without checking and stay out of the house | Something will catch on fire – 80% belief |
| | I will get so anxious (100%) that I will freak out and run down the road. It will last until I go back and check that everything is okay – 90% belief |

**COMPLETE AFTER THE EXPERIMENT**

| Did predictions come true? | Conclusions | Does this fit best with Theory A or B? |
|---|---|---|
| No | I think that things are more unsafe than they really are | This fits best with Theory B |

| Did predictions come true? | Conclusions | Does this fit best with Theory A or B? |
|---|---|---|
| Anxiety after 5 minutes, 90%; anxiety after 20 minutes, 80%; anxiety after 40 minutes, 50%; anxiety after 50 minutes, 30%; anxiety after 70 minutes, 10% | The anxiety was very unpleasant, particularly at the at the point where I thought a fire might be burning but it did go down and I didn't 'lose it' | I didn't know if I could handle the anxiety. This shows that I can, so it fits best with Theory B and tells me what happens if I try to act according to Theory B as well |

It is possible that for you it may take a few goes to build up to leaving the house without checking at all. You don't need to worry about this – recognise that this is very normal if you have been in the habit of checking excessively for some time. Any reduction in checking is good and is an achievement. However, you need to test out Theory B as much as possible and continue to progress towards the clearest experiment, in this case not checking at all and leaving the house.

## DON'T STOP THERE!

Once you have started kicking OCD out of your life, if you possibly can, really go for it. For Jennifer this would be repeating this experiment, going out for longer, doing it at different times and in different moods. There are several reasons why this is a good idea:

- Building up evidence for Theory B – it isn't just a fluke that Jennifer's house didn't burn down, she wasn't 'lucky this time' – she took a 'risk' and found out how the world really works.
- Reclaiming your life – OCD has held you back and taken things from you. Take pride in standing up to the problem and being free to do what you want to do. You do not need to live in OCD's dictatorship where there is a ban on socialising – do what you like and go out when and where you please.
- Protect yourself against future wobbles – if you have a bad day in the future then you can think back (and refer back to your notes) and remember that you did all these fantastic things to overcome your problem. (More on this in Chapter 9, Life After OCD.)

Once you have done this experiment, you need to do it again. The more times you have experienced the reality of what happens, the more evidence you will have stored to answer the intrusive doubts and thoughts that the OCD may fire off at you. Remember the anxiety extinction curve in the last chapter? When people repeat the experiments their predictions, and/or their belief in their predictions often change. In parallel with this, the intensity of the anxiety they experience in the situation does not usually get as high and goes down more quickly. But please don't take our word for it. It is very useful to keep your own information on this by filling out the record sheets as it is often very hard to remember exactly what we thought and felt in the past. If you find the anxiety is not subsiding as predicted by Theory B, have a look at the troubleshooting section on page 180.

## DOING THINGS THE ANTI-OBSESSIONAL WAY

The key to breaking free as quickly and as thoroughly as possible is to do things in an anti-obsessional way. This could mean not checking at all and going out for a long time or practising letting the thoughts go when you get them, 'maybe I locked the door, maybe I didn't'.

## TACKLING BEHAVIOURS AND BELIEFS THAT KEEP A CHECKING PROBLEM GOING

Earlier, we identified some of the common behaviours and beliefs that keep a checking problem going. You will see how standing up to the OCD and not checking can challenge each one, and often several at the same time.

| SAFETY-SEEKING BEHAVIOUR | HOW IT KEEPS THE PROBLEM GOING | WHAT TO DO (BEHAVIOURAL EXPERIMENTS) |
|---|---|---|
| Checking things repeatedly | Keeps focus on danger and increases doubt. Undermines confidence in memory<br><br>Keeps you feeling anxious | **Don't check**<br>Rate belief in danger<br>Rate anxiety<br>Rate confidence in memory over several experiments |
| Asking for reassurance | Reassurance is a form of checking – it makes you feel less certain as you will always be able to pick holes in someone's answer | **Don't ask**<br>Rate belief in danger<br>Rate anxiety<br>Rate confidence in memory over several experiments |
| Avoidance | Avoidance means that the beliefs remain unchallenged. For example 'I cannot leave the house without checking' | **Don't check**<br>Rate belief in danger<br>Rate anxiety |

| ANXIETY-RELATED BELIEF | HOW IT KEEPS THE PROBLEM GOING | WHAT TO DO (BEHAVIOURAL EXPERIMENTS) |
|---|---|---|
| 'Once I've thought that something could go on fire, it would be irresponsible not to check' | To check is to be focused on danger. If you are checking, you will have more and more thoughts about danger. If you have to act on each one, you will soon find yourself doing lots more checking, thinking about more and more danger, doing more checking | **Don't check** Rate belief in danger Rate anxiety |
| 'I have a very poor memory' | Research shows that people with OCD do not have worse memories than others. However, doing lots of checking makes people less confident in their memory, a problem that they solve by ... doing more checking! | **Don't check** Rate confidence in memory over several experiments |
| 'I can't stop checking until I feel certain that things are safe' | Feelings are not a good way to make decisions like this. Checking makes you feel anxious, and anxiety makes you doubt and feel uncertain. Therefore it's easy to get stuck in a loop of trying to feel certain by checking, which makes you feel less certain, so checking more | **Don't check** Rate belief in danger Rate anxiety |
| 'Nothing bad has happened – the checking is working to keep me and others safe' | This is very seductive logic. But perhaps the checking is nothing to do with the fact that nothing bad has happened | **Don't check** Rate belief in danger Rate anxiety |

## CHECKING BEHAVIOURAL EXPERIMENTS:
TROUBLESHOOTING

*My anxiety isn't going down*

If your anxiety is not subsiding during the behavioural experiment, one of the more common reasons is that you may still be doing particular things to try to 'manage' the anxiety or prevent what you fear from happening. As we know, these sorts of things are what in themselves keep the anxiety and doubt going. So if your experience is that anxiety is not going down, ask yourself if there is any part of you that is acting as though the problem is one of danger when you are doing your experiment. For example, are you doing any mental checking by trying to remember if things were turned off in the house? Have you planned your experiment at a time that someone will be back soon to 'catch' a problem? OCD is a problem of doubt and fear. In a behavioural experiment, the more you can eliminate doubt that the reason nothing happened is because *it just wasn't going to anyway*, the more you will truly *know* that you don't need to follow the rules that OCD wants you to.

*Behavioural experiments are difficult; my problem is fine when I get someone else to lock the doors so I tend to do that*

It should be clear from reading this book that a broad sense of responsibility is a key thing that the OCD uses to get you to check. Often people will hold ideas such as 'I must do everything in my power to prevent bad things happening'. Therefore it follows that if someone else checks then they 'take on' this responsibility and that it is not your fault if something bad happens. This is a 'natural' example, but in therapy we may test this out more deliberately by writing and signing a contract to take responsibility for someone's house at a particular time on a particular day and ask them to monitor their anxiety before, during and after this time. The anxiety usually goes down at the point that responsibility is 'transferred'.

This is useful information as it fits very well with our understanding of the problem. However, in tackling it, you need to make sure that you *are* taking the responsibility at the same time as not doing everything in your power to stop what you fear happening. Not doing this is a form of avoidance that will keep the problem going, that is, your belief that the problem is danger and that you can't trust yourself. Of course, for some people, such as Jennifer, they find that they cannot allow others to check for them as they worry that others will not check to their high standards. OCD can go either way, depending on the individual person and circumstances. In both of these cases, the sense of responsibility is a key factor driving the OCD.

### It is very hard to ignore the thoughts of something bad happening

If this is the case it is important to remind yourself of what exactly these thoughts are. Remember that you are very tuned in to threat, as the OCD has made you feel very anxious. Anyone who is anxious has more anxious thoughts: that is just a normal part of being human. However, these are just thoughts, not premonitions or evidence that you must do something about them. In fact, if you do hold those sorts of beliefs about the thoughts, it is very important to find out what happens if you do *not* do something about them. In preparation, you can test out such beliefs in other ways, like trying to start a fire just by thinking about it.

## THE FUTURE: WHAT HAPPENS IF YOU CONTINUE TO TREAT THE CHECKING PROBLEM AS ONE OF WORRY?

Once you have done some behavioural experiments you should be able to see that the evidence points in one direction – that the checking OCD has been bullying you into believing that there is a lot of danger around. If you really accept that the problem you have is one of worry and fear, and live accordingly by acting against your fears, we predict that the anxiety will over time decrease and you will be able to reduce your checking. After all, you will have shown yourself on several occasions that it is possible to do things differently. Now you can incorporate that into your life and begin to do some of the things that OCD has stopped you from doing for so long.

Jennifer's first goals were to be able to leave the house without checking and to reduce the amount of time she spent checking. Once she began to do this, she was able to plan more extensive trips to do things she had not been able to do for a long time. Jennifer began to gain confidence – she stopped checking what her flatmates were doing and stopped asking them for reassurance, a very welcome change. As she had so much more time and felt better Jennifer was able to reconnect with her other friends and began to be invited out again, sometimes at very short notice – this helped her get her life back as well as providing opportunities to continue her fight against OCD. Jennifer was able to re-enrol on her university course and began to rebuild her life without OCD.

## BREAKING FREE FROM CONTAMINATION FEARS

In the previous chapter we looked at how an OCD problem of contamination develops and what keeps it going. We looked at the example of Suse, who became concerned about contamination with disease and whether she would cause harm to herself and other people. Over time her life became increasingly dominated by hand-washing, checking, asking for reassurance and other safety-seeking behaviours. Rather than making her feel better, these all served to fuel her obsessional belief that she would get ill and die (Theory A) and maintained her anxiety. Suse considered the alternative belief about her problem: it is a problem of anxiety about dirt and germs. Her Theory A/B table is below:

| THEORY A: OCD SAYS | THEORY B: OCD IS |
|---|---|
| The problem is that I will get contaminated with dirt, germs or disease and die | A problem of worry that I will get contaminated with dirt, germs or disease and die |
| **Evidence:** | **Evidence:** |
| People die from MRSA in hospital | I have often worried about things in the past |
| | I have read a lot of magazine articles about diseases that have made me worry more — it is actually very rare for people to catch these diseases and die |
| **If this is true, what do I need to do?** | **If this is true, what do I need to do?** |
| Wash my hands at least 50 times a day; use alcohol gel and wet wipes | Ignore thoughts about disease |
| Wash hands until they 'feel right' | Treat worries as worries — not as signs of imminent danger |
| Use anti-bacterial spray several times a day on all surfaces | Freely touch things when out in public without washing my hands |
| Keep on the lookout for brown or red marks on objects | |
| Ensure that I don't spread germs or disease to others | |

| If I keep following these rules, what will happen in the future? | If I keep following these rules, what will happen in the future? |
|---|---|
| *I will need to do more and more cleaning and checking; this will take over my life* | *I can do what I like with my life* |
| **What does this say about me as a person?** | **What does this say about me as a person?** |
| *I'm vulnerable* | *I am sensitive and I have a worry or anxiety problem but I am no more vulnerable than anyone else* |
| | *I am a determined person who wants to tackle this problem* |

## WHERE TO START?

Suse saw that her extreme caution and avoidance and all her washing had not helped her; it had made her problem worse. The solution had become the problem. However, she still felt quite strongly that the risk from disease was very high but she decided to try to act as if Theory B were true ('fake it till you feel it'). She realised that she would need to touch things that she would usually avoid and not do any of her safety-seeking behaviours – no hand-washing, no alcohol gel, no touching things through gloves or tissues, no trying to 'track the spread' of contamination. She was worried that she would feel really anxious for a very long time but bravely decided to find out if it would be as bad as she thought. Particularly important … she gave up all thoughts of undoing any of the behavioural experiments she was doing. She was particularly surprised when she noticed that as she stopped keeping track of contamination, she felt very much better. She came to realise that this was because she was no longer preoccupied with ideas of going back and cleaning those things she had contaminated. To do this, she had completely committed herself to the idea of Theory B ('my problem is being worried'), which helped her focus on fighting her true enemy rather than endlessly and pointlessly trying to get rid of contamination.

## SUSE'S BEHAVIOURAL EXPERIMENT

**COMPLETE BEFORE THE EXPERIMENT**

| Planned behavioural experiment | Specific predictions and how much I believe them |
| --- | --- |
| Go on the bus and touch the door on entry and exit; touch the seats and poles several times | I will feel 100% anxious for the whole day and will not be able to function |
| | I will get flu (belief that this will happen: 100%) |
| | I will be hospitalised within 24 hours (80%) |
| | I will pass flu to Tony (90%) |
| | He will be hospitalised within 24 hours (90%) |
| | I will die (50%) |
| | Tony will die (60%) |

**COMPLETE AFTER THE EXPERIMENT**

| Did predictions come true? | Conclusions | Does this fit best with Theory A or B? |
|---|---|---|
| Anxiety ratings before going on bus: 90%<br>On bus: 95%<br>Touching pole: 95%<br>Touching door: 95%<br>20 minutes later: 70%<br>1 hour later: 40%<br>2 hours later: 15%<br>24 hours later: 0%<br>Did not get flu<br>Did not pass flu to Tony<br>Did not die<br>Tony did not die | I did feel very anxious at the time but actually it passed very quickly as I was not doing any of my safety behaviours. Neither Tony nor I was ill in any way. I noticed that no one else on the bus seemed that bothered about touching it. If other people can be so relaxed on the bus, I can too | This fits best with Theory B. My safety-seeking behaviours have not made me safer — I didn't do them and nothing bad happened. Theory B tells me to treat my horrible thoughts about disease as just thoughts — when I did this I still felt anxious and uncomfortable but I was able to behave as others do and had the opportunity to learn what happens when I don't avoid things |

## DON'T STOP THERE!

Once you have started kicking OCD out of your life, if you possibly can, really go for it. For Suse, that would mean going on several more buses (that day if possible) and touching the door as much as possible (and not washing her hands afterwards).

There are several reasons why this is a good idea:

- Building up evidence for Theory B – it isn't just a fluke that Suse didn't die from touching the bus door. She wasn't 'lucky this time' – she took a 'risk' and found out how the world really works.

- Reclaiming your life – OCD has held you back and taken things from you. Take pride in standing up to the problem and being free to do what you want to do. You do not need to live under OCD's dictatorship where there is a ban on bus travel – do what you like and go everywhere that you please.

- Protect yourself against future wobbles – if you have a bad day in the future then you can think back (and refer back to your notes) and remember that you did all these fantastic things to overcome your problem. (More on this in Chapter 9, Life After OCD.)

## DOING THINGS THE ANTI-OBSESSIONAL WAY

For Suse to really build up her confidence and kick the OCD bully out of her life, she decided to take her bus behavioural experiment into 'anti-obsessional' territory. She repeated her bus journey, but this time she took food with her and ate it after touching several parts of the bus interior. She deliberately touched a seat that she saw someone else touch – so she knew for sure that she was in contact with potential contamination from others.

> Suse felt very anxious on the bus but touched several parts of the interior, making sure that she did not sneakily avoid touching any particular bit of the bus. When she saw another passenger touch the pole she deliberately touched that bit. She thought, 'What am I doing! I might as well let him spit in my face!' – then she reminded herself that OCD had made her a prisoner in her own home and made her miserable for such a long time. She grabbed the pole again and then ate her sandwich. She felt nervous but at

the same time elated. When she got home she had a few horrible thoughts about disease but tried to let them go without monitoring herself for signs of illness. She touched her phone and diary when she got home – to 'spread' the bus contact. She then got on with a job application and realised she hadn't thought about the bus journey for some time, and that she did not feel anxious at all. The next day she had a phone call from a friend asking her if she wanted to go for an impromptu picnic – she was delighted to accept, knowing that she could cope.

## TACKLING BEHAVIOURS AND BELIEFS THAT KEEP A CONTAMINATION PROBLEM GOING

Earlier, we identified some of the common behaviours that keep a contamination problem going. You will see how standing up to the OCD and not doing all your washing, avoiding and so on allows you to find out what happens – how the world really works. You can also find out if you do feel as anxious as you predict.

| SAFETY-SEEKING BEHAVIOUR | HOW IT KEEPS THE PROBLEM GOING | WHAT TO DO (BEHAVIOURAL EXPERIMENTS) |
|---|---|---|
| Washing hands or other body parts or inanimate objects in a repetitive ritualised way | Once lengthy washing starts, any shorter or less comprehensive washing doesn't feel 'enough'. Rituals and repeating don't make things any cleaner; the only result is feeling more anxious | **Don't wash** Did your predictions come true? Did anything bad happen? Were you as anxious as you predicted, for as long as predicted? |

| SAFETY-SEEKING BEHAVIOUR | HOW IT KEEPS THE PROBLEM GOING | WHAT TO DO (BEHAVIOURAL EXPERIMENTS) |
|---|---|---|
| Using how your hands 'feel' to work out when to stop washing | This is a dangerous way to decide to stop washing; the more anxious you feel, the more you feel dirty, the more you wash, the more anxious you feel ... | **Lick hands or touch other people with hands that 'feel' dirty** Did your predictions come true? Did anything bad happen? Were you as anxious as you predicted, for as long as predicted? |
| Avoiding touching, e.g. door handles | By avoiding, you prevent yourself from finding out what would happen if you do touch all these things – that actually you are unlikely to contract a disease or spread it to anyone else | **Don't avoid** Did your predictions come true? Did anything bad happen? Were you as anxious as you predicted, for as long as predicted? |
| Being on the 'lookout for trouble' e.g. looking for red or brown marks, monitoring yourself or other people for signs of ill health | This is a form of selective attention; once you start looking, you will spot marks on objects that no one else would have seen. By throwing the objects out, ('better safe than sorry') you do not have the opportunity to find out that the marks on the objects were harmless. By tuning in to whether anyone is showing signs of ill health, you will notice the smallest sniff or cough | **Pick up objects with red or brown marks** Did your predictions come true? Did anything bad happen? Were you as anxious as you predicted, for as long as predicted? |

All your behavioural experiments help you challenge your beliefs about being responsible for preventing something bad happening:

| ANXIETY-RELATED BELIEF | HOW IT KEEPS THE PROBLEM GOING | WHAT TO DO (BEHAVIOURAL EXPERIMENTS) |
|---|---|---|
| I am responsible for preventing the spread of contamination/dirt/germs and stopping something bad happening – illness or death | No one can actually stop the spread of all dirt/germs/disease. All your efforts to try to reduce the risk actually focus on the potential danger and lead to you feeling more responsible, not less | **Don't do any safety-seeking behaviours** Did your predictions come true? Did anything bad happen? Were you as anxious as you you predicted, for as long as predicted? Re-rate your belief |
| If there is and risk that something is dirty/contaminated, I must do something about it | By not taking the risk, you don't get to find out that actually nothing bad happens | **Don't do any safety-seeking behaviours** Did your predictions come true? Did anything bad happen? Were you as anxious as you predicted, for as long as predicted? Re-rate your belief |

## CONTAMINATION BEHAVIOURAL EXPERIMENTS:
TROUBLE-SHOOTING
*But what if I die at some indeterminate point in the future
from touching the bus door?*

> *Suse was really pleased with herself for going on the bus
> for the first time in years. She was able to go out to see her
> friend Tony whom she hadn't seen enough recently. The
> day after, she actually forgot about her worries and
> realised she hadn't been thinking about whether she had
> flu or not. Then she had a horrible image of Tony dying
> and had a nasty feeling that maybe she had contaminated
> him with a deadly disease that would lurk in his body for
> a few years without symptoms before making him horribly
> ill. She realised that she could not be 100% sure that this
> would not happen and felt very anxious.*

Not all OCD beliefs can be tested with a single experiment. Suse
was able to find out that touching a bus door did not lead to her
immediate death but there is no way of testing out the prediction
that she or Tony would die in the future. What Suse needed to do
was 'tolerate uncertainty'. She could not be absolutely sure that
there was not a deadly disease on the bus; no one using a bus can
have this certainty. Despite feeling anxious, what Suse needed to
do was ignore her thoughts about Tony dying and not take any
steps to try to feel less certain or to reassure herself.

*I'm not anxious; I feel disgust when thinking about
touching something dirty*
You might find yourself curling your lip in disgust, or feeling angry
that other people have been careless in a public toilet. In those
situations, take a moment to think about what is so bad about it?
If all you feel is disgust for a short while, that is common and not

a concern. However, if you 'carry' the feeling of disgust with you for hours or days afterwards, and take measures to get rid of it through washing, or avoiding situations in the first place – then ask yourself 'If it's disgusting, so what?' It is possible that there is another idea lurking in there; perhaps that you will transfer germs to other places, get ill or never be able to get rid of the disgust feeling. Behavioural experiments will be useful for challenging these beliefs. Research shows that disgust subsides when people confront their fears.

## When I get physically dirty I feel mentally dirty too

In Chapter 2, we described 'mental contamination' – the feeling of inward pollution or being dirty on the inside. Recently, psychologist Professor Jack Rachman, pointed out the link between feelings of mental contamination and important formative experiences: it seems that we can feel contaminated and dirty because we have been *treated like dirt* when we were trusting. This feeling is dealt with by attempts to wash away the feeling; because the feeling is inside, the washing fails, of course. Discussing these issues with a therapist will be useful (see Chapter 7). As described on page 48, for some people it can be helpful to make the link between past events and the internal feeling of 'pollution', in order to understand why washing is in fact of no use. Having clearly made that link, treatment follows the same pattern as described in the rest of this book, including developing a 'vicious flower' and carrying out behavioural experiments to test out the relative value of Theory B versus Theory A. Theory B will tend to take the form of 'My problem is that past events made me feel dirty/violated/ betrayed and this has made me wash too much even although I am not dirty ...'. As noted above, often working in this way requires help from a therapist who specialises in OCD, so that you can work with them to build up your understanding of the problem and then use that understanding to overcome the OCD.

## THE FUTURE: WHAT HAPPENS IF YOU CONTINUE TO TREAT THE CONTAMINATION PROBLEM AS ONE OF WORRY?

Once you have done some behavioural experiments you should be able to see that the evidence points in one direction – that the contamination OCD has been bullying you into believing that there is a lot of danger around and that you are responsible for preventing something bad happening. If you really accept that the problem you have is one of worry and fear, and live accordingly by acting against your fears, we predict that the anxiety will, over time, decrease and you will be able to abandon your obsessional ways. Once you take courage and do some behavioural experiments, you can find out for yourself that it really is possible to do things differently. Now you can incorporate that into your life and begin to do some of the things that OCD has stopped you from doing for so long.

> *Suse looked at her goals for the future – she wanted to start dating and get into a relationship and get a job. She had found both of these difficult as she had so little time to do anything other than washing her hands and she had avoided going out. Now that she had learned how the world really worked, she was able to go out and meet people, and go to job interviews. She was able to make applications for all sorts of jobs without worrying about whether the work place would be 'contaminated' in some way.*

# BREAKING FREE FROM INTRUSIVE THOUGHTS AND RUMINATION OCD

In the previous chapter, we looked in detail at the processes and reactions that keep a rumination problem going. We considered the problem as one of many vicious circles operating at the same time which fuel a sense that the thoughts are meaningful and important (Theory A) and thereby keep the anxiety going. We have been looking at the example of Jeremy, who began to engage in a number of behaviours that fuelled his central belief that he was a potential danger. The more that he 'bought in' to this idea and acted accordingly, the worse and more severe his rumination problem (and belief in Theory A) became. It was suggested to Jeremy that there was an alternative way of thinking about his problem, that it was one of extreme anxiety about danger (Theory B) and that his measures to try to manage danger had actually served to make his anxiety worse. Jeremy completed his Theory A/Theory B form.

| THEORY A: OCD SAYS | THEORY B: OCD IS |
|---|---|
| The problem is that I might harm my daughter | The problem is I worry that I might harm my daughter |
| **Evidence:** | **Evidence:** |
| The thoughts make me feel very anxious | Feeling anxious is not evidence that I will act on the thoughts. The fact that the thoughts make me feel anxious means that I do not want to act on them |
| **If this is true, what do I need to do?** | **If this is true, what do I need to do?** |
| I can't take a risk – check myself for any signs I may act on the thoughts | See the thoughts as just thoughts and carry on with what I want to do with my life |
| Avoid contact with my daughter | Don't avoid anything – do more of it in fact |
| Avoid contact with all children | |
| Push the thoughts away or try to cancel them out | |
| **What does this say about the future?** | **What does this say about the future?** |
| This will be hard and difficult to maintain. To be safe I will stay away from others | The future looks good |

| What does this say about me as a person? | What does this say about me as a person? |
|---|---|
| *I am a bad person* | *I am a caring, sensitive person* |

## WHERE TO START?

It is important that you identify the particular reasons that you think that, in your case, the thoughts are important, dangerous, or mean something bad about you as this will help you plan experiments to test out these ideas. For Jeremy, one of the ideas that kept him anxious was his belief that the sheer amount of thoughts he was having meant that he was closer to losing control. As a result he was trying to control his thoughts in various ways such as pushing them out or reassuring himself and thinking 'good' thoughts. He tried not to control his thoughts to test the impact on his beliefs and anxiety and to try to shed light on whether having more thoughts meant that he was more dangerous.

## JEREMY'S BEHAVIOURAL EXPERIMENT

### COMPLETE BEFORE THE EXPERIMENT

| Planned behavioural experiment | Specific predictions and how much I believe them |
|---|---|
| *Alternate between controlling the thoughts as much as possible and trying not to control them on different days* | *When I don't try to control the thoughts I will get too many of them to handle* |

| Planned behavioural experiment | Specific predictions and how much I believe them |
|---|---|
| *Try to count thoughts and rate anxiety* | *I will feel very anxious, 100%* |

**COMPLETE AFTER THE EXPERIMENT**

| Did predictions come true? | Conclusions | Does this fit best with Theory A or B? |
|---|---|---|
| Day 1 (controlling): Lots (hundreds) of thoughts as usual. Anxiety 80% all day Day 2 (not controlling): I still got the thoughts but fewer over the day and my anxiety went from 80% in the morning to 30% by afternoon. I think I started thinking about other things! Day 3: as day 1 Day 4: as day 2 | Engaging with the thoughts and controlling them makes them seem more real and makes me feel anxious. I also get many more. Trying to control them has actually made me less in control as I haven't been able to do what I want | This fits with Theory B, where my worry about the meaning of the thoughts makes me react and gives importance to the thoughts and I feel more anxious |

## DON'T STOP THERE!

Once you have started kicking OCD out of your life, if you possibly can, really go for it. For Jeremy, this meant fully letting go of trying to control the thoughts. Jeremy really tried to stand up to the OCD bully. He made every effort to stop asking for reassurance and when he caught himself arguing and trying to 'prove' to himself that he was not a bad person, he decided to say 'well maybe I am a bad person!' and went and did something else, like playing with his daughter.

Why is this such a useful thing to do to break free from OCD?

- Building up evidence for Theory B – it isn't just a fluke that Jeremy did not act on his thoughts when he stopped controlling them, he wasn't 'lucky this time' – he took a 'risk' and found out how the world really works.
- Reclaiming your life – OCD has held you back and taken things from you. Take pride in standing up to the problem and being free to do what you want to do. You do not need to live in OCD's dictatorship where there is a ban on socialising – do what you like and go out when and where you please.
- Protect yourself against future wobbles – if you have a bad day in the future then you can think back (and refer back to your notes) and remember that you did all these fantastic things to overcome your problem. (More on this in Chapter 9, Life After OCD.)

## DOING THINGS THE ANTI-OBSESSIONAL WAY

Jeremy courageously decided to go a step further and actually deliberately bring on the thoughts in 'risky' situations in order to test things out as fully as possible.

---

**COMPLETE BEFORE THE EXPERIMENT**

| Planned behavioural experiment | Specific predictions and how much I believe them | |
|---|---|---|
| Try to bring on the thoughts and images of harm | I will lose control and hurt the baby | Anxiety level |
| 1. when near the baby | 60% | 100% |
| 2. when holding the baby | 80% | 100% |
| 3. when holding a knife near the baby | 100% | 100% +++ |

---

**COMPLETE AFTER THE EXPERIMENT**

| Did predictions come true? | Conclusions | Does this fit best with Theory A or B? |
|---|---|---|
| 1. I felt very very anxious doing this – 100% for 20 minutes, which then went down to 20% after another 20 minutes | I was very anxious about my thoughts when near the baby | I am definitely someone who worries about their thoughts |
| 2. Anxiety went up to 80% but came down after 20 minutes | This experiment really challenged my beliefs that thoughts could make me lose control and I found that even though I was very anxious I was nowhere near losing control | This experiment shows that I don't act on them, even when I am getting them a lot |
| 3. Anxiety went to 80% but came down after 15 minutes | | |
| I did not hurt the baby | | |

He took what felt like a huge risk in bringing on his feared thoughts in a situation where he felt he was more likely to act on them. In doing this he really left the OCD nowhere to hide – he now knew that even by acting in an anti-obsessional way, which made him feel very anxious, he was still not going to act on his thoughts.

The more you can act in an anti-obsessional way, the less space the OCD will have to convince you that the reason nothing happened was because of luck, or some special circumstance that happened.

# TACKLING BEHAVIOURS AND BELIEFS THAT KEEP RUMINATION AND INTRUSIVE THOUGHTS GOING

| SAFETY-SEEKING BEHAVIOUR | HOW IT KEEPS THE PROBLEM GOING | WHAT TO DO (BEHAVIOURAL EXPERIMENTS) |
|---|---|---|
| Mentally reviewing events | This is a form of checking. It keeps focus on danger and increases doubt. Undermines confidence in memory. Keeps you feeling anxious | **Don't go over things** Rate belief in danger Rate anxiety Rate confidence in memory over several experiments |
| Thought suppression | Trying to suppress thoughts makes you have more of them. In order not to think of something, you need to think of what it is you are trying to push away | **Test this out** by trying to suppress other thoughts like a 'polar bear' (see page 72). Compare supressing with not supressing |
| Asking for reassurance | Reassurance is a form of checking – it may give you temporary relief but ultimately makes you feel less certain as you will always be able to pick holes in the answer | **Don't ask** Rate belief in danger Rate anxiety |
| Avoidance | Avoidance means that the beliefs remain unchallenged; as you are 'acting as if' it is true, your obsessional belief feels more true | **Go into situations you have avoided.** Try to 'lose control' by bringing on thoughts |

| ANXIETY-RELATED BELIEF | HOW IT KEEPS THE PROBLEM GOING | WHAT TO DO (BEHAVIOURAL EXPERIMENTS) |
|---|---|---|
| Thinking something is as bad as doing it | This means that thoughts are themselves a source of danger – it is impossible to not have these thoughts | **Go into situations you have avoided.** Try to lose control by bringing on thoughts |
| I am a bad and dangerous person or I wouldn't be having these thoughts | Because you are worried about being bad, you are on the lookout for 'bad thoughts'. Therefore you will notice every thought that fits with this idea and you will generate more of such thoughts. If this seems like 'evidence' then the belief will strengthen. This is a vicious circle | **Ask** a trusted person if they have ever had thoughts like this. Several research studies show that most people experience 'intrusive thoughts' |
| In order to feel safe, I need to be completely certain that I won't do something wrong | It is impossible to achieve a sense of certainty about obsessional doubts. The more you try to be certain the less certain you will feel, and so you will get stuck in a vicious circle | **Go into situations you have avoided.** Try to lose control by bringing on thoughts Practise 'tolerating uncertainty' Did your predictions about how bad it would be come true? Were you as anxious as you predicted, for as long as predicted? |
| The thoughts I have mean something fundamental about me | This belief will drive you to try to work out what the 'true' meaning of the thought is | **Ask** a trusted person if they have ever had thoughts like this. Several research studies show that most people experience 'intrusive thoughts' |

| ANXIETY-RELATED BELIEF | HOW IT KEEPS THE PROBLEM GOING | WHAT TO DO (BEHAVIOURAL EXPERIMENTS) |
| --- | --- | --- |
| Anxious thoughts can damage my brain | This is, of course, an anxiety-provoking thought and is an OCD trap. We are all hardwired to be able to experience anxiety and when it is in proportion it is a useful and necessary thing  Anxious thoughts cannot be damaging. OCD is unpleasant and stressful and in this way can damage you by keeping you anxious for long periods of time | Do a survey – do other people experience anxious thoughts? Has it damaged their brains? |

## RUMINATION AND INTRUSIVE THOUGHTS BEHAVIOURAL EXPERIMENTS: TROUBLESHOOTING

*I feel irresponsible for 'accepting' my bad thoughts*

You may *feel* very irresponsible and reckless by acting in this way – this is one of the ways that the OCD has bullied you. It is not irresponsible and reckless to stand up to a bully, far from it. What you are doing is experiencing for yourself the way the world really works. The OCD may even have convinced you somewhere along the line that you can't trust your judgement or who you are. This is what it wants you to believe so it can stay around, 'advising' you on what to do to stay safe. Very much like a bully, it has stopped you from seeing how things work for yourself and has undermined your confidence. Keep rebelling against this unhelpful friend and you will soon enough get your confidence back and put the thoughts back in line with all of your other thoughts.

## THE FUTURE: WHAT HAPPENS IF YOU CONTINUE TO TREAT THE RUMINATION PROBLEM AS ONE OF WORRY?

Once you have done some behavioural experiments you should be able to see that the evidence points in one direction – that the rumination OCD has been bullying you into believing that your thoughts are dangerous or mean something bad about you. If you really accept that the problem you have is one of worry and fear, and live accordingly by acting *against* your fears, we predict that the anxiety will, over time, decrease and you will be able to reduce your rumination. Now you can incorporate the fact that this is a problem of worry into your life and begin to do some of the things that OCD has stopped you from doing for so long.

> Jeremy really grasped the nettle and acted as though Theory B was true, although at times he did not feel this. However, by doing this he stopped avoiding and over time his intrusive thoughts reduced significantly and he began to believe and feel that he was a good enough person. To his wife and the rest of his friends and family he was already a fantastic person but they noticed how much happier he seemed. He no longer avoided any of the tasks he needed to do as a parent and found that he was much more present in all that he did.

# BREAKING FREE FROM RELIGIOUS OCD

Johnson had drawn out his Theory A/B and knew that his blasphemous thoughts were no different from millions of other religious people. He realised that OCD had made him very focused on his thoughts and he had become so preoccupied with what he was thinking that it had become a 'self-fulfilling prophecy': every time he picked up his Bible he thought 'I hope I don't get any of those horrible blasphemous thoughts' – and so he did. He realised that he was stuck in an OCD trap and he needed to really embrace Theory B to escape.

| THEORY A: OCD SAYS | THEORY B: OCD IS |
|---|---|
| The problem is that my thoughts are blasphemous and I will be condemned for them | The problem is that I am so committed to my faith that I have worrying thoughts which seem blasphemous, so I fear that I will be condemned for them |
| **Evidence:** | **Evidence:** |
| It is a sin to have sexual images when you are in church or thinking about God | The images are not things I have chosen to think about and they make me feel very anxious |
| | I have always tried to live a very Christian life and there is no other evidence that I am a bad person. I worry about this because I am religious |
| **If this is true, what do I need to do?** | **If this is true, what do I need to do?** |
| Try to push the thoughts out of my mind | Ignore the thoughts |
| Look out for the thoughts | Not monitor my thoughts or my body |
| Try to atone for them at every opportunity | Go to church and study the Bible regardless of any intrusive thoughts |

| | |
|---|---|
| Avoid situations where the thoughts could be triggered | Not avoid anywhere or anything |
| Stay away from church | |
| **If I keep following these rules, what will happen in the future?** | **If I keep following these rules, what will happen in the future?** |
| I will need to do more praying and avoiding; this will take over my life | I will have a closer relationship with God and my church |
| **What does this say about me as a person?** | **What does this say about me as a person?** |
| I'm a bad person | I am a religious person, who takes their religion and morals very seriously |

## WHERE TO START?

Recruiting a friend or family member to help is often extremely helpful. It can feel very risky explaining the problem to someone else, but most often it brings great relief to everyone. We will discuss this in greater detail in Chapter 8. Family and friends almost always notice that there is something wrong, even when you try to hide your OCD – finding out what is troubling you is usually better for them than constantly worrying and trying to guess what is going on. Most people with OCD find that family and friends try to understand their concerns and desperately want to help. Show them this book and the work you have done linked to it to help them share your understanding of how OCD really works.

Johnson asked another member of his church, Hans, to help him with his problem. He explained that he'd had thoughts that he didn't want to have in church and that this had made him feel like he was a very bad person. Hans told him that his mind often wandered in church and he sometimes found himself think-ing things that he wished he had not. He told Johnson about religious figures from history who had suffered with this problem. Together they planned a behavioural experiment; Hans agreed to do everything that Johnson did.

Johnson went through the three choices. He was clear that the obsessional choice was to avoid his church and Bible and to try to suppress his thoughts. The non-obsessional choice was to ignore the thoughts and carry on regardless. The anti-obsessional choice was to bring on the thoughts in church or while reading his Bible. He understood that the anti-obsessional choice would be useful for several reasons and explained the Special Forces metaphor to Hans: it is useful to prepare yourself for difficult situations – if he practised bringing on the thoughts in church, next time it happened unexpectedly he would be prepared and know what to do. For example if a thought popped into his head during communion and his belief that he was a bad person became very strong, resulting in him wanting to leave, or actually leaving, the building, he would know that he needed to go back in and allow the thought to stay in his head and not to do anything else differently.

He agreed with Hans that they would both think about sex during the next service at church. Johnson predicted that he would then have many intrusive thoughts that he would find disturbing; he planned to ignore these thoughts, letting them come and go. Johnson's behavioural experiment was therefore an anti-obsessional choice.

## JOHNSON'S BEHAVIOURAL EXPERIMENT

### COMPLETE BEFORE THE EXPERIMENT

| Planned behavioural experiment | Specific predictions and how much I believe them |
| --- | --- |
| Going into church and having a thought about sex | I will be plagued with further thoughts about going to hell (100%)<br><br>I will be so anxious that I will make a fool of myself and feel more disgraced |

### COMPLETE AFTER THE EXPERIMENT

| Did predictions come true? | Conclusions | Does this fit best with Theory A or B? |
| --- | --- | --- |
| I did have a lot of other thoughts that I found disturbing but I stayed in the church<br><br>I did feel very anxious (50–60%) for most of the service but I did not make a fool of myself or feel disgraced<br><br>Several people came up to me to chat and once we got talking I found the thoughts easier to ignore and my anxiety went down to about 20% | Hans said that he had lots of other thoughts as well; he reminded me that most people would and that the thoughts are just thoughts. I have been trying to control my thoughts or avoid having thoughts in the first place and it has made me feel worse. This has been a real challenge for me; I have stood up to the temptation to give in to the OCD and I feel proud of myself. It was good to see my friends at church | This fits best with Theory B. When I treat thoughts as just thoughts my anxiety decreases and I feel better |

Earlier we identified some of the common behaviours and beliefs that maintain a problem of OCD about religion. You will see how letting the thoughts come and go or ignoring the thoughts is a key strategy in getting rid of the problem.

| SAFETY-SEEKING BEHAVIOUR | HOW IT KEEPS THE PROBLEM GOING | WHAT TO DO (BEHAVIOURAL EXPERIMENTS) |
|---|---|---|
| Trying not to think about it (thought suppression) | Suppressing thoughts actually generates more thoughts | **Let thoughts come and go** Did your predictions about how bad it would be come true? Were you as anxious as you predicted, for as long as predicted? |
| Trying to think about something else (thought substitution) | This is 'buying in' to the idea that the thought is significant and wrong and that it is necessary to get rid of it by substituting another thought – the original thought is likely to come back again, and more | **Let thoughts come and go** Did your predictions about how bad it would be come true? Were you as anxious as you predicted, for as long as predicted? |
| Selective attention – to thoughts or body parts | Being on the lookout for thoughts makes them more noticeable. Feeling anxious can lead to many changes in bodily sensations; by paying attention to his genitals he guaranteed that he would notice some changes | **Let thoughts come and go; don't monitor body** Did your predictions about how bad it would be come true? Were you as anxious as you predicted, for as long as predicted? |

| Rituals – e.g. praying for hours to ask for forgiveness | Prayers become repetitive and prolonged and 'buy in' to the idea that it is wrong to have the thought in the first place. Trying to get the prayer 'right' can bring on more of the intrusive thoughts and images and fresh doubts about your faith | **Don't do rituals** Did your predictions about how bad it would be come true? Were you as anxious as you predicted, for as long as predicted? |
| Avoiding religious practice | By avoiding activities that are consistent with observance of of your faith you may feel more upset and guilty and your belief that you are bad can feel more believable and true | **Don't avoid** Rate anxiety Did your predictions about how bad it would be come true? |

| ANXIETY-RELATED BELIEF | HOW IT KEEPS THE PROBLEM GOING | WHAT TO DO (BEHAVIOURAL EXPERIMENTS) |
| --- | --- | --- |
| Having this thought means that I am a bad person | Your values and religious beliefs might mean that you are more likely to interpret an intrusive thought as significant and meaningful – but everyone has intrusive thoughts | **Let thoughts come and go** Were you as anxious as you predicted, for as long as predicted? Re-rate your belief |
| I should be able to get rid of these thoughts | It is normal to have intrusive thoughts, images or doubts – it is impossible not to. Trying to get rid of the thoughts actually makes them more noticeable and treats the thoughts as important | **Let thoughts come and go** Were you as anxious as you predicted, for as long as predicted? Re-rate your belief |

## Religious OCD behavioural experiments: troubleshooting

### I can't bring myself to do it, it feels so wrong

Remember that we all have cultural, moral or religious values that govern behaviour; the idea that we are violating these values or rules 'feels' very powerful and frightening. Step back and think whether what OCD makes you do really does fit with your true beliefs and values.

### Won't I be going against God by doing the behavioural experiments and stopping my rituals?

This is an easy one. No matter what your religion, there is *no way* that God wants people to suffer OCD at all, let alone a type of OCD that gets in the way of you having a good relationship with God. God wants you to serve Him through love, not to feel constantly terrified. If you could ask, God would pretty much certainly say, 'Please get rid of your OCD so that we can have a better relationship.'

### How can I be sure that I am not going to go to hell?

Discussing your problem with a clever and compassionate leader of your faith can be very helpful. Remember to focus on building up your evidence for Theory B – that this is a problem of anxiety and worry. Remember how OCD has taken away your ability to practise and enjoy your religion – this bad thing has already happened.

## The future: what happens if you continue to treat the religious OCD problem as one of worry?

Once you have done some behavioural experiments you should be able to see that the evidence points in one direction – that the religious OCD has been bullying you into believing that there is something wrong with you, or that you are a bad person and that there is something dangerous going on in your thoughts. If you really accept that the problem you have is one of worry and fear, and live accordingly by acting against your fears, we predict that the anxiety will, over time, decrease and you will be able to abandon your obsessional ways. Once you take courage and do some behavioural experiments, you can find out for yourself that it really is possible to do things differently. Now you can incorporate that into your life and begin to do some of the things that OCD has stopped you from doing for so long. Our experience is that once people stop having to do loads of rituals to make sure that they have not blasphemed or offended God, they are able to develop a much more positive approach to their faith.

---

*Johnson looked at his goals for the future – he really wanted to go on a trip with his church friends. He had been scared to do so as he thought he would be consumed with intrusive thoughts and would not be able to leave when he wanted. He decided to sign up for the trip and started to look forward to it. When he went, he found that he did have some difficult times when he found himself thinking blasphemous or sexual thoughts. Another person noticed he was quiet at these times and asked him if he was okay. Johnson told her that he had some problems with anxiety and worry and that sometimes he found it harder than other times. She offered him sympathy and support. As the trip went on Johnson found he was spending far more time enjoying himself than he was thinking about OCD.*

# BREAKING FREE FROM OTHER TYPES OF OCD

As should be clear from this and previous chapters, everybody is different and unique, and everybody's OCD is also different and unique. However, it is possible to categorise the focus of OCD in a number of ways; for example, washing versus checking, thoughts of having done something potentially harmful versus thoughts that a harmful thing *might* happen. We have already explored the fact that people with contamination fears can be worried about contamination by germs, by poisons or even by places or people linked to bad memories. There are similar variations in other 'types' of OCD. It should come as no surprise, then, that some people suffer from OCD symptoms that do not easily fall into the 'categories' discussed so far in this book. So does this mean that if you have an 'unusual' form of OCD, you won't be helped by CBT and the ways of applying it discussed in this book? Good news! The answer is that you *will* be helped.

You will see from reading the last few chapters that whatever form of OCD you have, OCD works in the same way and uses many of the same tricks to keep itself going. This is very important information as OCD can sometimes be there in more than one form or can change over time. We have guided you through our detailed case examples from understanding of how OCD became and remained a problem, to how the person used this knowledge to get rid of the OCD bully and get their life back. The basics of breaking free from other commonly encountered types of OCD are the same, with the details being different. In each case, an alternative, worry-based explanation needs to be identified and tested out. A key part of testing it is to carry out behavioural experiments to confirm that the problem is one of worry and, where possible, to discover that not only does anxiety and distress decrease, but also it may be possible to discover that the things you fear will not happen. In any event, it will always be possible to discover that the discomfort decreases and will disappear if you are able to stop ritualising.

Some examples of other types of OCD fears include:

- I worry that something bad might happen if I don't avoid unlucky numbers/cancel out my thoughts/follow a ritual
- I'm worried I've hurt someone without knowing it
- I feel very uncomfortable if things are not in their right place
- I'm worried I may be gay/straight and in denial

## TROUBLESHOOTING: ROADBLOCKS TO MAKING PROGRESS

### I UNDERSTAND HOW OCD WORKS, BUT WHAT IF MY PROBLEM ISN'T REALLY OCD?

OCD is a very idiosyncratic problem and can be focused on almost anything that the person finds dear or important to them at that time. What this actually is, of course, varies from individual to individual.

OCD is sometimes known as the doubting disease. One particularly toxic doubt that can go along with having OCD is whether your particular problem truly is OCD. If you have had this doubt, you may have read the last few chapters thinking something like, 'I understand that, but *my* form of OCD doesn't quite fit'. The implication of your problem not being OCD is that the original meaning that the thoughts you have is true, i.e. you are still being sucked into Theory A, the idea of danger. If you treat the thought 'What if I do not have OCD?' as an intrusive doubt then you can draw a vicious flower based on this which might look something like the following:

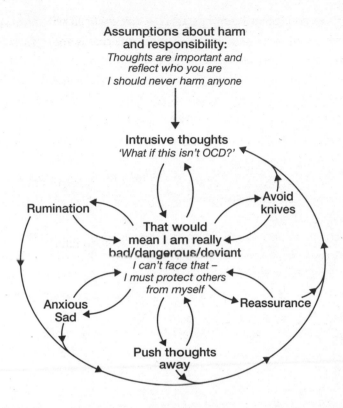

## I can't accept that I'm not really dangerous or bad

This is a related issue that people can come up against. Remember that until now you have spent a lot of time trying to protect others from harm, as it has felt safer than risking the tiniest doubt that what you fear may be true. It's worth really thinking about that – consider not only what sort of person worries about thoughts and harm but what sort of person spends so much time and effort trying to prevent themselves harming others? Is it really the sort of person whom you would think of as dangerous or bad? With whom are you comparing yourself? You might be thinking about the 'worst in society', murderers or paedophiles, or people who have suddenly 'lost the plot'. Sometimes people with OCD are concerned that they may be like people who act on thoughts of harm. In many cases, the only point of comparison is that they also had thoughts of harm. Unfortunately, most people who carry out terrible and horrific crimes did not worry about their thoughts of harm, nor did they spend lots of time and effort trying not to do bad things. The majority of people have occasional thoughts of harm which they may find a bit unpleasant but they are not bothered by these.

Perhaps you are bothered by things in your past that feel like they mean something definitive about you. If you think of someone you really define as 'good' do you think that this person has never offended anyone or done anything even slightly 'wrong'? It is unlikely. In fact at any time in life, but particularly when we are young, we can make all sorts of 'mistakes', as we are learning about the complexities of other people and about ourselves. Most people will have done things that they would go back and change at least some detail of, if they had a time machine. The point is we all do some things wrong and our negative feelings about these things can help us ultimately be better and not make the same mistakes again. Is it possible that you are judging things in your past from the point of view of having all the information at hand? It may be that you developed ideas about yourself from negative experiences while growing up. Please see the Resources section on page 269 for information and books that can help more with general issues underlying OCD.

## I can't be sure that it's Theory B, so it's safer to act as though it is Theory A

This relates to the discussion above: the OCD has been telling you that it is better to be safe than sorry. This would be fine if those were the options you were actually choosing between. The fact is that OCD comes at an immense cost to yourself and your family and is a very unsafe option, as it damages lives. It's important to really think about this and engage with the reality of what OCD is doing and could do to your life. Even if OCD has taken a huge amount from you, the good news is that you can decide to do things differently and get your life back.

## I'VE DONE SOME EXPOSURE BUT I'M STILL ANXIOUS

If your anxiety is not subsiding during the behavioural experiment, one of the more common reasons is that you may still be doing particular things to try to 'manage' the anxiety or prevent what you fear from happening. As we know, these sorts of things are what in themselves keep the anxiety and doubt going. So if your experience is that anxiety is not going down, ask yourself if there is any part of you that is acting as though the problem is one of danger (Theory A) when you are doing your experiment. For example, are you doing any mental cleaning when you are touching something contaminated? Have you planned your experiment at a time that someone will be back soon to 'catch' you in the act if you did something wrong? OCD is a problem of doubt and fear. In a behavioural experiment, the more you can eliminate doubt that the reason nothing happened is because *it just wasn't going to anyway*, the more you will truly *know* that you don't need to follow the rules that OCD wants you to.

Outside the experiments, have you really *lived* according to the idea that it's a worry problem? It's important not to hold back because doing that is what is keeping you anxious.

## I'M NOT GETTING RID OF THE PROBLEM AS FAST AS I WANT

It's good to move as quickly as possible to overcome your problem but do not beat yourself up if you do not achieve your aims as quickly as you want. You might find yourself 'automatically' washing your hands in certain situations, or you might find your intrusive thoughts and anxiety harder to ignore than you anticipated. Be kind to yourself – you are tackling a difficult problem. Being hard on yourself, calling yourself names or criticising yourself, is never helpful when trying to overcome OCD. Calling the OCD bully rude names is to be encouraged! Also you might want to consider enlisting the help and support of someone you trust; overcoming OCD is a tough prospect, and it is really helpful to have someone to cheer you along and pick you up if you stumble.

If you do slip up, a great thing to do is to turn defeat into victory! People often find that the urge to ritualise or neutralise in some shape or form comes back from time to time, especially when they feel stressed (but also sometimes when they feel happy). OCD tries to get its foot in the door, and when you are at your most vulnerable. This is, of course, the best time to fight back to make sure that you are completely on top of the OCD. For example, almost without thinking, when you have touched something contaminated, you wash. An intrusive thought, image, impulse or doubt pops into your head; before you know where you are you have argued or neutralised it. You check the door several times when you are trying to get out of the house in a hurry. Now, this is not out of control but is an example of an old habit reasserting itself, rather like the ex-smoker reaching for their cigarettes. Habits and tendencies of this type need to be actively counteracted once you notice they are happening.

So you washed after you felt particularly contaminated when you touched a sticky door handle? Go back and contaminate your-self even more than you were in the first place! Touch the door handle again, or find something that seems even more contaminated as an act of defiance. Spread that contamination!

You checked the door? Unlock it again, leave it unlocked then walk five minutes up the road and five minutes back, then lock it and *don't check*.

Had a blasphemous thought in church and then begged God for forgiveness? Get a couple more of those blasphemous thoughts into your head, then get on with the ceremony, hymn or prayer that is going on once you have got the un-neutralised thoughts in your head.

You went out of your way to avoid doing something? Go back and do it!

In summary, once you have got rid of most of your OCD but still have little urges to ritualise, avoid or put things right in an OCD way, listen carefully to the small but insistent voice of OCD which remains, and *do exactly the opposite of what it says*. Go 'over the top' if you can.

Don't give OCD house room or a foothold. Push it so far out of your life that it can't come back.

# 7

# CHOOSING TO CHANGE

The previous chapters have discussed how OCD can start, how it keeps going and how you can apply that understanding to move on and break free from OCD. Sometimes, simply having this knowledge is not enough; you are doing your compulsions for very particular reasons. It is important to remember what is at stake as, now you have some knowledge about OCD, how it works and the consequences, sticking with the OCD and not changing is an active choice. In this chapter we will talk more about helping you choose to move on from your OCD, and how to find and get the best out of professional help if you need it.

## GOALS
In Chapter 3 we asked you to think about your goals by reflecting on what the problem has taken from you and what you would like to do if you did not have this problem. We have spoken a lot about how you might start to go about changing and beating the OCD. Now is a good time to have a look at your goals again to remind yourself of why you want to go through the difficult process of breaking free.

## PROS AND CONS OF CHANGING
It should be clear that people begin to fall into obsessional patterns of thought and behaviour, not because of doing something wrong, but because this is the only choice they have with the understanding they have at the time. A number of background factors can also play a role in the development of OCD. Without

it being a person's fault, or even their choice, OCD then develops as the best coping mechanism available at the time and it can feel like it works, or did work to some extent, which is a very powerful maintaining factor. But as we know, over time it becomes the problem, keeping people locked in its world of fear and safety-seeking. Sometimes, the initial sense that OCD helped to cope with a difficult situation can remain. It is not uncommon to fear whether you can cope with difficulties once you let go of your obsessions and compulsions.

If this sounds familiar, then it is worth thinking systematically about whether or not you really want to live without OCD. Write down on a piece of paper the advantages and disadvantages of being obsessional. What are the advantages and disadvantages of not being obsessional? Often this will help clarify the issues, as in the example of Jennifer (checking OCD) below.

| ADVANTAGES OF BEING OBSESSIONAL | DISADVANTAGES OF BEING OBSESSIONAL |
|---|---|
| Helps me 'feel' safe | Really I feel anxious all the time |
| | I don't go out |
| | I don't have any friends |
| | All I think about is danger and checking |

| ADVANTAGES OF *NOT* BEING OBSESSIONAL | DISADVANTAGES OF *NOT* BEING OBSESSIONAL |
|---|---|
| I could be 'normal'! | I might be less careful |
| I could go out and meet people | (although this doesn't mean I would be careless) |

Consider, as we did when thinking about Theory A and Theory B, the short-term and long-term effects of continuing with the obsessional behaviour versus becoming non-obsessional.

We have already used the metaphor of an insurance policy to think about the price of 'safety' that the OCD is selling you. Perhaps a more apt version of this is that OCD is really like a protection racket! The problem comes in, creates an atmosphere of fear and danger and then offers to help 'protect' you from the danger if you follow the OCD rules. The danger is very much coming from the OCD itself, and following the rules will cost you dearly.

As an exercise it really is worth thinking ahead a few years to what it would be like if you continued to be obsessional and to follow the rules that OCD has set for you. Imagine it's the 21st birthday party of the eldest child of a mother with obsessional concerns about keeping her children safe and the child reads out the following speech:

> *Firstly, thank you all for coming to my 21st birthday party. Thank you friends and family but mostly thank you, Mum, for keeping me alive until now. I know that this must have been a difficult task due to the many many hours that you put into it since I was born. It is a shame that this left you too exhausted to play any games with me in the evenings, but I know that you were doing your best, and as I say, I am grateful to be alive. It might have been nice to be allowed out once in a while to play with the other children or have them over, but I realise that the threat this presented to me must have been a very great danger. Of course I knew that when you shouted at me to wash my hands it was because you were worried about my safety and this helped me learn that these things were very important for survival. As I say, the proof is that I'm here now.*

Think through all the areas that OCD is affecting in your life. There could be an alternative to this picture if you change what you are doing and live according to the idea that the problem is Theory B. Think it through; that birthday speech could read:

> *Firstly, thank you all for coming to my 21st birthday party.*
> *Thank you friends and family, but mostly thank you, Mum,*
> *for being so loving and so courageous in dealing with your prob-*
> *lems. I know that this must have been a difficult task due to*
> *the many many hours that you used to spend on it. It was great*
> *that you had more and more time to do stuff with me, and it's*
> *so fantastic that despite your anxiety you always let me out to*
> *play with the other children or have them over when I wanted.*
> *I didn't know at the time what you were going through, but*
> *I'm proud to now. My girlfriend says I'm a very sensitive and*
> *caring person which must be down to you, so thank you.*

# PROBLEMS THAT PEOPLE EXPERIENCE DURING RECOVERY AND HOW THESE CAN BE OVERCOME

## ROCKING THE BOAT

If you have made some progress it can be tempting to think 'that will do, why risk going any further? Why rock the boat?' At the start of tackling your problem you thought yourself to be in a tempestuous sea in a tiny boat with no paddles – it would be foolhardy to rock the boat! However, now you have started tackling your problem, you can rock the boat – you can step out into a warm, shallow, tropical sea and head off to the land. In fact, it is important that you *do* rock the boat to find out that there are no limits in getting OCD out of your life and that you are able to do whatever you want without it. Rock the boat – then get out of it!

## RE-INFECTED WOUND

Maybe there is one last bit of OCD you can't imagine tackling. It is tempting to think that it is okay to have 'just a bit' of OCD.

You know only too well that if you give OCD an inch it will take a mile. Imagine if you had a nasty infected wound on your arm. Your doctor gives you antibiotics and it clears up – apart from one little bit. What will happen to the wound? It will become re-infected. The same risk applies with the little bit of OCD you might want to hang on to – your hard-won gains may be lost. OCD is not helpful or a friend and, because it is a horrible bully, it will always go back on a 'deal' and take more from you than you want to give it.

## WHEN SELF-HELP ISN'T ENOUGH: GETTING PROFESSIONAL HELP

It goes without saying that OCD is a tricky problem to beat and can be difficult to combat on your own, even with a good under-standing of how it works and the principles of how to move forward. Everyone is unique, and it is not possible in this book to describe all of the different ways in which OCD can trap you, and all the different ways that might be helpful when you are trying to overcome OCD. OCD sometimes 'disguises' itself, tricking you into thinking you are doing something helpful when in fact it is making things worse. It's worth doing the scale on page 20 every month to track whether your efforts are making the difference you hope for. If you graph month by month it should show a decrease overall. If you are trying your best and it's not making the differ-ence you hope for, *don't blame yourself.* Even with plenty of knowledge and understanding, OCD has defeated many people. Sometimes, you just can't do it on your own and need thought-ful support and expert guidance which links the principles set out here with your own unique pattern of reactions. This is the reason that it is a problem treated by trained and specialised therapists across the country. A body of experts and people who have expe-rience OCD have put together clinical guidelines for The National Institute for Clinical Excellence (NICE) regarding OCD and how best to treat it, based on a careful and detailed review of the exist-ing evidence. In summary, the treatment of choice for both children and adults with OCD is Cognitive Behaviour Therapy (CBT), a form of talking therapy, including Exposure and Response Prevention (ERP). Many people find they also benefit with the additional support of medication alongside the therapy – Selective Serotonin Re-uptake Inhibitors (SSRIs) are usually the medications of choice for treating OCD.

The website addresses are given in the Resources section (see page 269) so that you can read either the full guidance (which is not easy) or the version specially written for sufferers and carers.

If you do decide to seek expert help, please remember that your therapist will not do the hard work; as usual, that is up to you. Cognitive Behaviour Therapy can be thought of as a version of self help in which the support and guidance is offered by a therapist who can work with you to move through beating your problem and troubleshooting any difficulties as they occur. A good way of thinking about it is that it's like having a coach, trainer or teacher; you have to do the actual work, while the therapist's job is to help you understand what you need to do and work with you to improve what you are doing. As that process continues, you should begin to see what you need to do yourself … you become your own coach.

So how to get the treatment you want? Although attempts are being made to improve this, access to good-quality psychological therapy can be patchy, whether it is via the National Health Service or private therapy. Getting highly specialist help is particularly difficult. Here is some guidance on how to go about finding a therapist and how to get the most out of the treatment you are offered.

## FINDING A THERAPIST

Your first port of call should be the National Health Service. You are entitled to receive help with disabling and/or distressing health and mental health problems, and the NICE guidelines (see page 269) specify what that help should be: it is mainly Cognitive

Behaviour Therapy of the type described in this book. Go to your General Practitioner to tell them about the problems you have with OCD. This can be difficult, so maybe you might want to write a few notes in preparation for your visit. Summarise your problems at the moment, noting especially how these interfere with your life, what the OCD stops you doing and how it affects other people. Perhaps show them the results of the scale on page 20. Explain that you have tried self help (this book, and other things you have tried). Some people find it useful to print out the NICE guidelines or material on websites (provided by OCD-UK; see page 269) to show their GP what they might prefer in terms of possible treatments.

What happens next will depend on where you live, which can determine what services are on offer. You might be referred to a primary care therapist or a therapist working in a community mental health team or mental health unit. The best option would be referral to a Practitioner Clinical Psychologist or a nurse Cognitive Behavioural Therapist, but there are other types of therapist. We suggest that, whichever type of therapist you are offered, you should find out more about them, their training and preferred way of working (see below). Sometimes you might be offered treatment from someone who is a trainee; don't reject this out of hand because they are inexperienced. Check out whether they are being supervised, by whom, and how this is being done. If they are being supervised using audio or video recording (if that is something you feel comfortable with) and their supervisor is expert in OCD and CBT, then it is worth considering.

If you decide to seek treatment privately (paying for treatment outside the NHS) you need to be even more careful. NHS care providers are required to follow evidence-based guidelines as set out by NICE; private practitioners are not. With a myriad of OCD treatments available and online offers of quick-fix cures for OCD, you need to be careful about what is actually on offer and whether it is worth the money you will have to pay for it. Following news that the BBC found that even a cat is able to be registered with a regulatory body of hypnotherapists (see http://news.bbc.co.uk/1/hi/8303126.stm) we decided to suggest what people can do when trying to find a therapist not only privately but in the NHS.

The following sections offer guidance on choosing the right therapist, advice on how to get the most out of therapy once you begin it and maintaining the therapeutic relationship when things go wrong.

When choosing a therapist, especially if paying to go private, it is important to ask some relevant questions to allow you to gauge if your therapist is suitable and is qualified to be treating you. You can introduce this by saying that, before committing yourself to therapy, you would like to know a bit more about the therapy and your therapist. (After all, you would do the same thing with any other expert service you obtained such as a gym coach, or even a plumber). Hopefully, you won't need to ask many of these questions 'out of the blue' because the therapist will inform you about themselves and what they offer. If they don't, however, you should ask them which of the questions below you think important.

We know that doing this can be difficult, as you might feel embarrassed about asking questions which sound challenging, so you could consider taking this book along to your therapist as a way of introducing this topic, and show him or her this page. You can say Paul, Fiona and Victoria, who know a thing or two about treatment for OCD, strongly suggest that you do this. No therapist worth seeing will refuse to answer a few questions.

## THE QUESTIONS:

- What type of treatment will you be offering me?
- Have you had specific training in using CBT for OCD, including supervised practice? Do you still receive some supervision? (Supervision is a good thing ... Victoria, Paul and Fiona receive supervision on their work.)
- How long will treatment take?

The therapist should answer **'Yes'** to most of the following questions:

- Have you done much treatment for OCD before?
- Will we set out a specific CBT treatment plan just for me, including a 'shared understanding' (see page 129)? (Rather than the therapist using the same approach for every OCD sufferer.)
- Will goals be set together? (Rather than therapist setting the goals for you.)
- Do you use techniques called 'graded exposure' and 'behavioural experiments'?
- Do you intend, as therapy progresses, to set practical exercises or 'homework' for me and help me understand these exercises?
- Where behavioural exercises are set for homework, a really good pro-active therapist will, if necessary, even come to your home or the place of the exercise to do the exercises with you; are you able to do that if things get difficult?
- Do you provide cognitive and behavioural treatment, rather than just behavioural treatment, with the point of helping me understand how the problem works so that I can better work on it?

A good therapist will not mind you asking these questions and, in fact, any reluctance to answer these questions should in itself be enough to make you question if they are the right person for you.

Another factor when searching for therapists is to check their credentials and qualifications, but don't be fooled by the fancy letters after a therapist's name. If the therapist has loads of letters it's worth checking on the web what they mean. There are many official-sounding counselling and therapy bodies, but not all check the credentials of their members, so do your research and never be afraid to ask questions. We primarily recommend using therapists accredited with the British Association for Behavioural and Cognitive Psychotherapies (BABCP) which is the lead organisation in the UK for CBT therapists (not to be confused with the BACP).

Although there are more than 7,500 members of the BABCP, only about 1,500 are accredited, so when searching for a CBT therapist it is important to check they are 'accredited' members of the BABCP, or they are registered with another legally recognised body such as the Health Professions Council. Therapists need to meet strict criteria to become accredited by the BABCP. These include being a member of a specified core profession, following minimum training standards and having a sustained commitment to the theory and practice of cognitive and behavioural therapies. This ensures that all accredited CBT therapists have achieved a high level of competence in cognitive and behavioural methods, which has also been independently verified.

The BABCP is also responsible for the accreditation of all 'High Intensity' CBT courses which are being set up under the Government's 'Improving Access to Psychological Therapy' programme (IAPT).

The BABCP website (www.babcp.com) allows you to search their database of accredited therapists, click the 'find a therapist' link, which will then take you to www.cbtregisteruk.com. From there, you simply select obsessive–compulsive disorder in the 'choose a condition' field, and enter your postcode or town details. It is important to remember that, even with BABCP accredited therapists, you must still probe them, perhaps with the questions we suggested above, to check that they are a therapist with required knowledge and expertise to treat you.

## QUESTIONS TO ASK ABOUT QUALIFICATIONS

What is your professional background? Are you professionally registered with the Health Professions Council, Royal College of Psychiatrists, British Association for Behavioural and Cognitive Psychotherapy? (Hint … you can look up registration or accreditation for these bodies on the web.)

How long ago did you qualify? If a long time ago, how do you keep up to date with new developments?

## SUMMARY: THINGS TO LOOK FOR IN THE RIGHT THERAPIST

- Someone you can trust or believe that you can come to trust
- Someone who can respect you, and you can respect in the same way
- Someone who is good at therapy and helping people to make changes
- Someone who knows how to avoid the most serious pitfalls (usually this means someone who is trained, preferably with experience in treating OCD)
- Someone who keeps up to date with new developments

# HOW TO GET THE BEST FROM THE HELP THAT YOU ARE OFFERED

Okay, so let's suppose you have found a qualified therapist who you think you can work with and who is offering good-quality CBT. There are things you can do to get the best out of the therapy. This is important, because not only do you want it to go well but you want to get through it as quickly as possible.

## PREPARATION FOR TREATMENT

Prepare a brief timeline and history of your problem; make a very brief summary, possibly as a diagram, on when things started to be a problem, when they got worse. Note on it any major events in your life (marriage, death of a loved one and so on).

It can also be helpful to summarise the main ways in which the problems impact on your life.

## ONCE THERAPY STARTS

- If your therapist doesn't usually do this (many do), ask if it is possible to record therapy so that you can go over it after the sessions. A good way to do this is to keep a notebook in which you write between five and ten things that you learned from the session, and at the back make a note of things it would be helpful to clarify with the therapist when you next meet them.

- In general, writing things down can help, either as notes for yourself or to hand to the therapist.
- Ask for things to read.
- Make sure you are on time, and don't miss sessions.
- Be aware of things which you find difficult to discuss. Try to decide not to keep important secrets (once comfortable with your therapist). OCD likes secrets! Perhaps make a list of things you find difficult to discuss, also writing (or saying) why it is difficult if you know why (for example, because you are embarrassed, because you are afraid that saying things might make them come true, because you fear that the therapist will think you are a bad person and so on).

## SHARED GOALS

Quite early in therapy your therapist should discuss what the goals of therapy are and how these match with your longer-term goals, which include what you want for yourself and your family in years to come, and what has to happen for these to come about. Many of the therapy goals can be linked to this; if you want to do a training course, first you have to be able to leave your house and feel comfortable going to other places, for example.

## GUIDED DISCOVERY

Your therapist will want to ask you a lot of questions about the problem. Some of these will be obvious questions about what life is like for you day to day. Some of these questions will be to gain a shared understanding where your knowledge about the problem is married with your therapist's knowledge of how obsessional problems work. As treatment progresses, your therapist will ask you questions that will help you to weave new information and ideas into your thinking, to help you to make the big changes you need to make to get rid of the problem. Remember, your therapist is probably something of an expert in anxiety, OCD and its treatment, but you are the expert in your life and the way OCD affects you, so in therapy you need to work closely with your therapist as a kind of partnership of two experts learning from each other about your problems and how best to tackle them.

## QUESTIONNAIRES

Your therapist will give you questionnaires to complete quite regularly. Do these (and, if appropriate, discuss them with the therapist) These are a good way of keeping track of progress both in general terms by totalling the scores and, more specifically, your therapist will often keep an eye on specific items or the pattern of change for clues as to what is happening.

## HOMEWORK

CBT therapists will almost always suggest homework, so that you can consolidate what you have learned between sessions. This might be reading, keeping records of specific events, 'behavioural experiments' where you gather new information about how your problem works by trying things out and recording the results. There are some key points that you should understand before you leave the session about homework, especially behavioural experiments. Often when the homework is set these points are clear, but pay attention to make sure that you understand:

1. Why are you doing this? What do you hope to learn from it?
2. How will you do it? When will you do it? (Try not to leave it to the day before your next session.)
3. How will you record the results?

When you have your next session, try to make sure that you put the homework on the agenda so that you can get the most out of understanding what you did and what it meant.

People suffering from OCD tend to be perfectionistic: make sure that you are doing the homework in the way that makes the most of what you can learn from it. Being perfectionistic and worrying about whether you did the work correctly is a sure-fire way of missing the point.

Again, this is best dealt with by making sure that there is a clear rationale for homework, always to be agreed between you and reviewed next session.

If you feel overwhelmed at the prospect of any homework suggested by your therapist, they will prefer that you say so and that you discuss what it is that concerns you. If you simply can't do it, again tell your therapist so that they can help you find another way of achieving the same objective which is, of course, to better understand and manage your problems.

## OTHER CLAIMS OF SPECIAL OCD TREATMENT METHODS

Occasionally you may also come across websites for individual therapists or private clinics that claim to provide a specialist treatment service that they may have developed differently from traditional Cognitive Behavioural Therapy. It is worth remembering that the treatment of choice for OCD is Cognitive Behavioural Therapy, the only psychological treatment shown to be effective, and therefore the only talking treatment recommended by the National Institute for Health and Clinical Excellence (NICE) based on a very careful review of the evidence which is, before being issued to the professionals and public, open for general discussion by all those who think that their particular approach has been ignored or treated badly.

It is also important not to allow yourself to be persuaded by these websites, many of which look highly professional and glossy with lots of testimonials from recovered sufferers – they are selling a service and therefore will not be providing independent reviews. Even respectable companies on the high street emphasise the positive feedback they receive and don't advertise criticisms.

You may also come across treatment methods written by people claiming to be ex-OCD and anxiety sufferers – don't assume that just because someone is an ex-sufferer, they are qualified to be a therapist to treat other people. So always, always, check the professional background and clinical training of the therapist/treatment method author.

Many of these treatment method websites and clinics also claim to be NHS approved; we have in the past seen examples of this where the authors' own GP had recommended the treatment method to another client, which was then being used to support claims of 'NHS approved'. Again, it is important to take these claims with a pinch of salt, and remember if these services were in fact fully NHS approved then they would be recommended by the National Institute for Health and Clinical Excellence (NICE) in the treatment guidelines for OCD.

## DISCLOSING SENSITIVE INFORMATION

For treatment to work it is important that you are open and honest with your therapist, no matter how strange or embarrassing your OCD may be: most therapists will have heard such stories before anyway so it won't shock them, as you had perhaps imagined.

Of course, with some forms of OCD about harming or abusing, especially children, it is naturally something that you will be afraid to tell anyone, and sadly not all health professionals have experienced these forms of OCD to be fully understanding, but please do not let this put you off seeking treatment.

What we recommend is perhaps to start out by talking about any other forms of OCD that you may have, and loosely touch on your harm OCD without going into specifics until such time as you feel you can trust your therapist, and your therapist is showing some understanding of the problems you are experiencing. Chances are, when you start touching on the subject of harm, the therapist may well understand what you are referring to and will help you express your fears, making you feel much more relaxed.

Should you have any problems expressing your OCD to your therapist, please do contact OCD-UK and they may be able to act as an independent intermediary for you.

## SO WHAT HAPPENS IF THERAPY IS NOT WORKING?

The therapeutic relationship plays a key factor in the success of a treatment – you and your therapist should be working and setting goals together and applying exercises as a team. However, even the most excellent of partnerships will sometimes slow down, and even hit the proverbial brick wall. In such situations it is important that you talk to your therapist, explain to them what you're feeling and thinking about the treatment progress. A good therapist should have spotted this in any case, either because it was obvious in sessions or because the questionnaires that you have completed show that all is not as well as it should be.

Communication is vitally important for therapy to work.

In situations where the treatment does slow down, talking to your therapist should help. New goals can be set, and new exercises planned together ('*together*' being the operative word). Beware the therapist that simply turns round and accuses you of not working hard enough – it is important to be honest with yourself and sometimes we may need to push ourselves a little more, but invariably if a therapist mentions a lack of investment on your part, then this is the sign that a new partnership may be needed. You can ask yourself if you are doing your best; if the answer is 'No', then of course you need to ask your therapist to support you in dealing with that. If, as is usually the case, the answer is that you are indeed doing your best, it might be that the therapist is not skilled enough, or even that their way of working and personal style does not match well with what you need. Seeking referral to someone else, usually with more specialist expertise, would be a helpful thing to discuss in a positive way.

Although we always suggest talking problems through with your therapist first, if you really feel your therapy partnership has gone as far as it can, there is nothing wrong with searching for a new therapist. That is not the sign of failure; it may just be that a new approach is needed. Think of it like learning to drive: you don't always pass your test first time and may need to try a different driving school. If you don't pass first time, you try again, and if needs be, again and again until such time as you're driving down the road to an OCD-free life.

# WHEN OCD IS NOT THE ONLY PROBLEM – WHERE TO GO WITH OTHER DIFFICULTIES

It may be the case that you are having to cope with other difficulties at the same time as OCD. Alternatively you may find that, as you start to tackle your OCD and that takes up less of your time and attention, other problems come to the fore and reveal themselves. It sometimes happens that in confronting OCD, it becomes apparent that the OCD has had the function of providing some way of coping with other difficulties, for example stopping you thinking about and dealing with a traumatic experience. When two or more problems occur together this is known as co-morbidity. The sections below give an overview of some common difficulties that can be co morbid with OCD and how you might think about tackling them with further professional or self help. Please also see the Resources section on page 269.

## HOARDING
Hoarding is the compulsive collecting of particular objects, to a level that interferes with daily life. People who hoard have immense difficulty throwing things away, often due to fears that they may accidentally throw away something of importance along with their rubbish or that the object may be useful in some way at a point in the future. This can be a very serious problem and the available living space can quickly become cluttered and unusable. In severe cases, compulsive hoarding can present risks to health due to being

a fire hazard. There is some debate as to whether hoarding is a form of OCD, with most professionals and researchers agreeing that it is a problem that may share some features and vulnerability factors with OCD but also has its own particular characteristics. Hoarding can be associated with OCD in that some of the reasons underlying the person's attachment to objects are due to fears that something bad will happen if they throw them away. This is similar to 'magical thinking' found in OCD in which people will perform rituals in order to keep themselves or others safe. Hoarding can also co-occur with OCD as a completely separate problem. Currently, hoarding is treated within services specialising in OCD. If you would like professional help with hoarding, you should approach your GP for a referral to a service treating anxiety disorders. It will be important that, as part of the assessment, the therapist visits your home (or where the problem is located) to get a sense of the extent and severity of the problem.

## DEPRESSION

Depression often results from having OCD. The level of restriction and interference that OCD causes means that the majority of people with OCD have secondary depression. It therefore follows that if the OCD improves, then so should the depression. However, for some people, depression is a problem in its own right, and even once they have got on top of their OCD they still experience symptoms of depression, or these symptoms can be so strong that it is very difficult to undertake treatment such as Cognitive Behaviour Therapy which involves actively thinking about and doing things. Symptoms of depression include depressed (low) mood for most of the day and nearly every day and loss of pleasure in things over at least a two-week period. Other physical symptoms may include changes in appetite, weight loss or gain, interference in sleep patterns and concentration, and feeling restless and irritable or very lethargic. Psychological symptoms may include thoughts and feelings of worthlessness and thinking about death a lot.

If you feel very depressed it can affect your motivation to do anything at all, even go out of the house. This is often associated with thoughts about your self-worth and assumptions as to how others may think of you and treat you. However, by not going out, you can reinforce these ideas, as you do not have any other information. A well-evidenced starting point to deal with depression is to plan some activities that, taken as a whole, provide you with some sense of pleasure and some sense of achievement and to do them, even if you feel like it is the last thing you want to do. There are several excellent self-help books that outline the cognitive behavioural approach to depression and which will guide you to use CBT to help you manage your mood and your feelings about yourself. However, if you feel suicidal you should tell someone that you trust and seek professional help to give you the support you need to get out of the depression.

## Generalised Anxiety Disorder

Generalised Anxiety Disorder (GAD) is the problem of having *excessive* and *uncontrollable* worry about a number of different topics for at least a six-month period. People with GAD will often have had the problem for much longer than this and may consider that they have 'always being a worrier'. GAD can be a very serious problem that can affect a person's sleep, appetite and ability to relax and so their life and ability to function in general.

GAD differs from OCD in that the topics that the person worries about don't clash with their values and they do not worry about what it means for them as a person to think about or not think about, or act, on these things. They are simply worried about bad things happening and the worry often jumps around from topic to topic. People with GAD get consumed with the content of their worries. The worrying is experienced as uncontrollable and is very unpleasant. Sometimes it is compounded by further fears that the worry is damaging to health and sanity, thereby causing further worry. This problem is thought to affect over 4% of the population and is treatable using Cognitive Behaviour Therapy.

## SOCIAL PHOBIA OR SOCIAL ANXIETY DISORDER

Social phobia is a severe fear of the reactions and judgements of others in social or social performance situations. It is quite a common problem affecting 7–13% of adults. People who suffer from social phobia experience a distressing amount of anxiety whenever they are in a feared social or performance situation. They are concerned that they will do or say something that will be humiliating or embarrassing. For example, they often fear that other people will see them blush, sweat, tremble or otherwise look anxious. Their fears may be general or specific to a few situations and due to their fears people with social phobia may avoid these situations or endure them with significant distress. The problem is at a clinical level if it causes significant interference in the person's life. Social phobia is treatable using Cognitive Behaviour Therapy even if you have had the problem for a very long time.

## AUTISTIC SPECTRUM DISORDER

Autistic Spectrum Disorder (ASD) includes autism and a milder form called Asperger's syndrome. The main feature of ASD is difficulties in 'social communication', that is the ability to understand the minds, intentions and feelings of others. People with autism experience problems with social interaction, communicative language and symbolic or imaginative play from an early age. The problem is one that is present from early childhood and persists through life, but the degree to which people have these problems can vary greatly. As adults they may avoid eye contact, use very few words, experience changes in routine as very anxiety-provoking and find metaphor very difficult. Most people with OCD do not have an ASD. However, research on people who do have these disorders shows that OCD or behaviour that looks like OCD is relatively common in that group. Only a trained specialist can make a clear diagnosis of an ASD in an adult or child and there are several national centres where such expertise is available. If you think you may have an ASD it might be worth exploring an assessment as this can help you access specialist help for any difficulties you may be experiencing, including OCD.

## PTSD AND EXPERIENCES OF ABUSE OR NEGLECT

Post-traumatic stress disorder (PTSD) is a persistent reaction to traumatic experiences in which the person felt afraid for their life, or their physical integrity was violated. Such experiences can vary from road traffic accidents to sexual abuse in childhood or adulthood and may have happened quite recently or a very long time ago. As a result of the trauma, the person experiences ongoing fear and may experience flashbacks, dreams or reliving of the event or events, or may find themselves afraid in situations that trigger memories of the event. These memories can be distressingly incomplete. PTSD may make the person feel very numb and detached from others and causes significant interference and stress. Occasionally, OCD can develop in the context of a trauma as a separate problem, as it can seem like a way that it is helping the person to be safe in what feels like a very unsafe world. If you think you have PTSD it is important to get specialist help for this problem which can be very effectively treated using Cognitive Behaviour Therapy. Treatment centres for traumatic stress or PTSD will be able to offer this; in the UK, referral to these services is made via General Practitioners.

Sadly, it is also reasonably common to have experienced other types of abuse and stress such as bullying or parental hostility and neglect that can lead to significant problems in self-esteem and self-worth. The meanings that people internalise about themselves from these experiences can be linked with developing difficulties such as depression, low self-esteem and social anxiety. These experiences are also common in people who develop OCD. If you are in treatment for one of these problems then it is often helpful to discuss these sorts of earlier experiences with your therapist as they may be able to help you gain new insight and understanding to enable you to move on from the current problem and from these past experiences. The self-help books shown on page 270 are also recommended.

## HEALTH ANXIETY

Health anxiety is a close cousin of OCD. People's concerns are about disease and falling ill at some point in the future and they frequently seek reassurance. This often results in concerns about contamination which can lead to excessive hand-washing and avoidance. Health anxiety is somewhat different from OCD, as a significant component of the problem is monitoring one's body for symptoms and trying to self-diagnose or seek diagnosis from health professionals. This problem can be treated with Cognitive Behaviour Therapy.

## BODY DYSMORPHIC DISORDER (BDD)

BDD is characterised by excessive concern about and preoccupation with a perceived defect in one's physical features. This can lead to extreme distress that interferes significantly with the ability to work, have relationships or even leave the house. Some people with BDD check their features repeatedly in a way that can resemble OCD but their underlying fear is not about responsibility for harm. This problem can be treated with Cognitive Behaviour Therapy.

## EATING DISORDERS

Eating disorders may occur with OCD and some of the features, such as avoidance or strict rules about eating, can overlap. However, beliefs about the importance of weight and shape are key aspects of eating problems that do not feature in OCD. The most common eating disorders are anorexia (the fear of being fat leading to being underweight and food restriction), bulimia (characterised by episodes of bingeing on large quantities of food and compensating by being sick, taking laxatives or excessive exercise) and binge eating disorder (when the person does not compensate for the binges). Eating disorders can be treated very effectively using Cognitive Behaviour Therapy which will help you look in detail at the beliefs and behaviours that are keeping the problem going.

## VOMIT PHOBIA

This is a severe and extreme fear of being sick. Vomit phobia predominantly occurs in females and is often a very long-standing problem. As a result of this fear, sufferers can alter almost every aspect of their behaviour. A common pattern is to avoid many foods and the feelings that some foods can give, in case these induce vomiting in the sufferer, to avoid particular places (such as bars, pubs, playgrounds and hospitals) due to a fear that the sufferer may encounter vomit in those places, or even to avoid certain people, in case these people may be sick themselves. As the range of possible situations where the person may encounter their fear is so broad, this phobia can be extremely incapacitating. Often, due to avoidance, and concern with things being clean, this problem can look like a form of OCD or an eating disorder, but it is driven by a particular fear of being sick or encountering vomit.

This problem is a recognised phobia which can be treated using Cognitive Behaviour Therapy.

# 8
# FAMILIES, FRIENDS AND OCD

This chapter is about the impact on those who live with or are close to someone with OCD and how these people may best try to help the sufferer through their difficulties. If you have OCD, there are sections on pages 27–31 and 257–260 for you to show your friends and family to help explain the problem and how they can support you.

Recent years have seen a much greater understanding of how the problem affects not only sufferers but also those around them including parents, partners, children and friends. We will talk about the various possible effects on others and how to minimise the impact on them, as well as maximising help from others when you are fighting OCD. Many types of relationships can be affected by OCD, but for ease of reference we will use the term 'family members' to include all of those who may be closely affected by the problem of another.

If you have OCD, or if you live with someone with OCD, you can probably think of instances where OCD has affected not just the person with the problem but others too. If you are stuck in obsessional patterns of thinking and behaving, this can affect other people and your relationships with them in a number of ways. It may be that you are frequently late for work or social engagements as it is taking so long to do rituals, which may be causing difficulties and stress with others. You may have started avoiding certain places or even people because to go near them would mean that you would have to be extra vigilant or you would have to spend a long time doing checking or cleaning at the time or afterwards. It may make things awkward or cause arguments if you are asking people to do things a certain way, or if you are preoccupied by your fears when you are with them. Perhaps you feel that others are simply better off or safer without you there and you may feel very down and not feel like mixing with people at all. Often people who have OCD get very good at making sometimes very subtle excuses for avoiding things or otherwise explaining their behaviour. However, after a point, other people may notice that something is wrong, even if they have no idea that OCD is the problem.

---

### COMMON WAYS THAT RELATIONSHIPS ARE AFFECTED BY OCD

- Getting other people to follow your obsessional rules
- Being irritable when others interrupt you during compulsions
- Asking others the same questions over and over again (seeking reassurance)
- Being late and changing arrangements because you are doing compulsions
- Avoiding certain activities, places or people because you will need to do compulsions
- Others worrying about you being so anxious

---

In some cases the fact that something is wrong can seem *more* apparent to others than to the person themselves as they are so consumed with their thoughts and rituals. This is because, particularly in the early stages of the problem, OCD can masquerade as a friend by offering the illusion of control and protection against danger. By its nature, OCD deflects attention from the bigger picture towards the moment-to-moment task of trying to feel safe. It can take a long while before people realise how much their life is revolving around the problem and just how much it has taken from them. Sometimes only a crisis, or a change in their lives that exposes the problem, can help people really face up to this. This is why it is really important to sit down and think about how much the problem is costing you, and those around you, before such a crisis occurs.

Because OCD is driven by the inner world of thoughts and interpretations, there are not usually many places that people with OCD feel genuinely 'safe' and free of the problem. If you are stuck in OCD, it is often going on in one way or another, most of the time. Therefore relationships are likely to be affected, as it is very difficult to hide the problem all the time, and the OCD is of course keeping you anxious and afraid. It can be very upsetting to see a friend or loved one being drawn into obsessional behaviour. This is particularly difficult when they cannot see themselves how destructive it is. OCD keeps people in a state of anxiety and alertness to threat, and the threat can be from internal sources (your own thoughts and feelings) as well as external sources (for example, contamination). It can be very difficult to make sense of for anyone who is not inside it, and it is difficult even if you *are* inside it. People with OCD are often told, asked or even begged by those that know them to 'just stop' their rituals and behaviours. Of course, if it were that straightforward, the person with OCD would have done this already. They may feel very frustrated in their efforts to stop ritualising and control the OCD. As the person with the problem, it can be hard to explain to others that, even though you know it is unlikely and even a bit irrational to think that something awful will happen, the fear of it happening is very powerful, particularly in the moment that it is triggered.

Often people will not disclose the contents of their intrusive thoughts even to loved ones, for fear that their reactions will confirm that they are somehow mad, bad or dangerous. Shame is a strong motivating factor for keeping OCD a secret, but it also keeps the problem going as people are left alone with their OCD fears and doubts with nothing to compare or reality check them against. If you have not told anyone in detail about your problem then, looking at this from the outside, the only information available to family members may be that you have become very anxious, secretive, avoidant, irritable or distant.

Even when they do disclose the problem to others, people are often torn between their anxiety and the knowledge that it is affecting their relationships. Feelings of guilt about the impact on others and worry that they are driving others away by their behaviour can further compound the problem. People can often feel terrible when they know their behaviour is having a damaging effect, but feel helpless to do anything about it. We will now have a look at some very specific ways that OCD behaviour gets in the way of relationships and how forces might be joined against the problem.

## Reassurance

One of the most common ways that OCD impinges on relationships is the need for frequent reassurance. As we discussed earlier, this is a very common means that people use to manage their anxiety. Asking someone to reassure you that the door is locked, that you didn't make a mistake or that you are not a bad person is a logical thing to do if you doubt yourself. However, when it is part of OCD it has the effect of keeping the problem going by reinforcing the belief that there is something to be reassured about, by raising more doubt and by undermining your ability to tolerate 'normal' uncertainty. Therefore, repeated reassurance seeking does not help the person, but helps the OCD.

Let's have a think about this again from the point of view of the person providing reassurance. By definition, to 'reassure' is to make certain *again*. This is an oxymoron, that is, the two parts of the word are conflicting, because if you were already certain, you would not of course need to do this repeatedly. For the person being asked to give reassurance this fact is plain, as they do not experience the anxiety, doubt and sense of over-inflated responsibility associated with OCD that drives people so strongly to look for certainty and safety. It can be very tiring to be asked the same questions over and over again if you cannot really see the point of it, apart from calming down the person asking you. Often, the reassurance becomes increasingly meaningless over time as the 'reassurer' will 'just say it' to try to satisfy the person with OCD. It is not uncommon for the person with OCD to be on high alert for this 'devaluing', as of course to them it is equally important each time and 'less than perfect' reassurance (as all reassurance is) will make them feel more anxious. They may feel *less* safe as they search for flaws in the reassurance, for example, 'He wasn't really paying attention then, how do I *know* he has cleaned the chicken and not touched anything else in the kitchen?' Such thoughts can lead the questioner to ask again, to monitor the behaviour of the other person, and to do the job again, but 'properly' this time. This can lead to tension, frustration and conflict with both parties feeling like they are not understood.

## GETTING OTHERS TO FOLLOW YOUR OBSESSIONAL RULES OR 'ACCOMMODATION'

This term was first used a few years ago to describe the degree to which family life is altered to adapt to or accommodate OCD. It makes sense that, if you are strongly driven to follow a set of obsessional rules, you may require others to follow these rules in order to stay safe, or to fulfil your sense of responsibility to keep others safe. After all, the OCD will not be satisfied until you have done everything in your power to protect others. This could be things like getting family members to check locks and appliances or asking them to wash their hands repeatedly or change their clothes as soon as they enter the house. Sometimes, it becomes difficult for the person with OCD to delegate any tasks as they just cannot be sure that others will carry them out with the same standards that they would have applied. They may become very anxious about sharing the tasks of family life and restrict what others can do or get into conflict about the standards of the people they live with. If the OCD is focused on the person worrying that they themselves are a danger then the opposite may be true, and they may want to delegate *all* tasks where they could cause harm. Given the nature of the problem, this can start to affect almost anything, for example food buying and preparation (fears of accidental contamination), driving (fears of accidentally running someone over) and childcare (fear of abusing a child). The avoidance that is so commonly found in OCD can affect the whole family in terms of the activities they are allowed to do, or the quality with which these things are enjoyed, and is, therefore, part of accommodating the problem.

---

**CASE EXAMPLE**

*Brian had been married to Mary for seven years. She had always been a scrupulous and careful person who kept things clean and in order but was able to enjoy life. Brian noticed that over time, her need for order and cleanliness began to become stronger and more rigid. They had always had a rule of taking shoes off when they came into the house but soon Mary required him to do this straight away and would become very agitated if he delayed at all. Before long she insisted he changed his clothes into ones she had washed for him as soon as he came in from work. The washing machine was constantly on the go. It became hard to have people round or to go out socially as Mary was very preoccupied with the idea that things outside the home could be dirty. This was very hard for Brian and while he tried to be understanding, he also felt resentful that everything in their life was affected by the problem. Things got particularly bad after they had their first child Jeff, when Mary became very preoccupied with cleaning and sterilising the baby's things. She insisted on performing all of the daily tasks for Jeff and would watch Brian carefully whenever he was looking after him. This led to many arguments and conflicts between them as Brian felt Mary did not trust him to look after Jeff. She*

> *would constantly ask Brian for reassurance that things were clean and that they had not touched anything dirty but would often go and clean them again anyway. Mary and Brian would often argue about this. Brian was often very sad to see that Mary had become so imprisoned by her anxiety, but felt that it was unreasonable that he had to follow her rules. However, if he did not, he knew that this could make her feel worse. He felt very stuck.*

Brian's story paints a stark picture of how OCD can affect a family. Clearly, in reality families are affected in a range of ways and to greater and lesser extents than this. People can get very good at compartmentalising the disorder, and as we know, people with OCD are very loving and caring and responsible. However, if OCD is affecting your family at all, then it is too much.

## HELPING YOUR FAMILY TO BREAK FREE FROM OCD

While we know that rituals, compulsions and reassurance make the problem worse, it is very difficult to deny help with these things to someone who is desperate and anxious. It is wholly understandable that families do give reassurance and even accommodate compulsions and rituals. The problem is not located in family members *doing* these things, but the fact that they are being asked to do them in the first place. If you have been doing this, then it is as a result of your OCD bullying you. Obsessional behaviour is born of fear. You do not need to feel guilty about it as you were trapped in this fear. Before you really understood what was happening and how OCD works you did not have a real choice to do anything differently; you were doing the best you could. Even knowing about OCD does not make it easy to change but it is certainly a good starting point. Now is the time to really get angry with this problem bullying you and getting in the way of your life.

The route to changing and breaking free from OCD is for *you* to understand the problem and what is unhelpful and to test out what happens if you do things differently. If you feel able, sharing this understanding and knowledge with a trusted loved one or friend can help in several ways. First, explaining the problem to someone else gives you a way to make sure that it makes sense to you and clarify your own understanding. If you would rather not explain in detail, you can talk in general terms about the principles involved, in particular the vicious flower we discussed earlier. Second, the other person may not really know about OCD, or about your OCD and what sort of a problem it is. It may come as a relief to know that this is a problem of anxiety that has a strong internal logic. Third, if the other person understands what OCD is and how it works, then they will better understand how to help you in your fight against the problem. Of course, only you can change your behaviour, but if you feel strongly compelled to avoid something, ask reassurance, or ritualise, they can help you focus on the fact that this is part of the OCD, not a behaviour that is keeping them or you safe, in order to help you in your decision making.

## SOME PRACTICAL STRATEGIES
- Explain how reassurance seeking and accommodation help the OCD by keeping the idea of danger going.
- Agree a form of words that your family member can use to remind you of that when you are anxious, e.g. 'It's just the OCD trying to have a go at you, it will pass.'
- Discuss with them how they can help support you when you are anxious and fighting the urge to ritualise, including when you want to seek reassurance. Ask if they might help by, for example, giving you a hug, putting on music or whatever you might find helpful as a way of coping with the anxiety of confronting your fears.

- Let them know of your goals and targets so that they can encourage and support you in changing.
- Don't worry about slip ups and giving in to the OCD if you do; recovery is not always a straightforward line, just try to learn from what happened and take each day as a new opportunity to take something back from the OCD. Similarly, your family should not worry if they 'give in' and give you reassurance or check something for you. See page 215 for more information about slip ups.

## BEHAVIOURAL EXPERIMENT: REASSURANCE

Mary would often ask Brian for reassurance. She would ask him if he thought that the bus was safe, if her hands were clean enough, if she had cooked food for long enough.

Mary and Brian discussed the role of reassurance – it makes OCD worse. Mary explained that whilst she experienced a temporary relief of anxiety, in the long term reassurance worked in the same way as all her safety-seeking behaviours – it made her thoughts and beliefs about contamination feel more important. It also made her reliant on other people – another way that OCD had robbed her of her freedom. Mary undertook to not ask Brian for reassurance but worried that she would get very anxious and might need to ask for it. Brian pointed out that refusing to give reassurance is hard and upsetting for both of them as he felt unkind and Mary would get upset. They agreed that rather than Brian refusing point-blank to give reassurance, he would try to remind Mary that reassurance is the OCD trying to ruin her life. They agreed that he would say:

- 'I think that's a reassurance question!'
- 'I will answer your question if you want me to, but can we remind ourselves about how this OCD works?'
- 'Do you remember this happened yesterday, and when I gave you reassurance you didn't feel any better, you ended up feeling worse?'

- 'You must be very anxious or you wouldn't be asking that question. Poor you. You are doing such a good job of trying not to ask questions – let's try to stick to it. What shall we do instead? How about a big cuddle?'

They agreed that Mary would cook dinner and try to not seek reassurance about whether the food was properly cooked:

| COMPLETE BEFORE THE EXPERIMENT | |
| --- | --- |
| **Planned behavioural experiment** | **Specific predictions and how much I believe them** |
| Cooking chicken for Brian | I will get the urge to ask Brian for reassurance (100%) |
| | I will need to ask Brian for reassurance (70%) |
| | Brian and I will get salmonella; symptoms will start within four hours (50%) |
| | We will be hospitalised within 24 hours (50%) |
| | Brian will die (40%) |
| | I will die (30%) |

**COMPLETE AFTER THE EXPERIMENT**

| Did predictions come true? | Conclusions | Does this fit best with Theory A or B? |
|---|---|---|
| *I did get the urge to ask for reassurance many times – when opening the packet of chicken, when taking it out of the pan, when eating. I did ask Brian when eating. Once when putting the chicken on the plate. He reminded me that it was unhelpful to answer. Neither of us got salmonella or died* | *The urge was there but I tried hard to overcome it and just have a normal normal conversation with Brian. I realise he usually gets stressed as I am always asking him questions – it was much better to just chat. I felt really anxious when I put the chicken on his plate and did ask him and he went through what we had agreed and we managed to not do actual reassurance. I felt very anxious for the first few minutes but I managed to ignore the urge and keep eating* | *This fits best with Theory B. I have been worrying about disease and making someone else ill* |

One of the best things about fighting back against your OCD is that it benefits not only you but those around you, and often straight away. You will have more time, more freedom and more clear-minded attention without this problem. A huge OCD lie is that not performing rituals and compulsions is irresponsible, and potentially harmful to others. It may *feel* like this at first, which of course does not make it true. If you ask your family, it is likely that they will agree that they do not get any benefit from you having OCD, and that they would rather have you back, OCD-free.

Mary felt horribly guilty about the impact of her fears on Brian but had always thought of it as doing her best to try to protect him and her son Jeff. While she knew she could go a bit far with her rules and worries, she had never really thought of it as a problem until she read an article on OCD in a magazine. This described many of the behaviours and thoughts she herself had. The more she thought about it, the more she realised that she had gone further and further in her behaviour which had had an effect on everyone in the family. Although they had not been physically ill for a while she understood that the home was not very happy. She showed the article to Brian who was hugely relieved to know that this problem had a name, and that treatment was available and effective. Mary researched OCD more and went to her GP who confirmed the diagnosis and referred her for CBT. During therapy she identified the problem as one of fear that she would be responsible for Jeff becoming ill rather than danger that he would become ill. She explained this to Brian, who was more understanding towards her not wanting him to help with Jeff. He was pleased that her goals involved not checking on him, and getting him to take Jeff out for the day, as well as allowing the house to become messy, well, less strictly neat and clean. He was particularly pleased that he no longer had to change when he came in. It was difficult for Mary in the first stages, and she would still frequently ask Brian for reassurance and would occasionally even clean after him. Although it was difficult to see the OCD bullying her occasionally, Brian was less annoyed as he understood why she did this. He felt *proud that she was confronting her fears that had been growing for so many years. The obvious delight of Jeff as Mary and Brian watched him play in the local sandpit was a strong motivator.*

If you are having difficulty not asking for reassurance or not asking others to follow obsessional rules, think about two visions of the future. Project forward to five or ten years' time. In the first exercise, imagine how family and social life will be if you carry on with the obsessional behaviour. Try to put yourself in the position of those around you and what their life would be like if they go along with it. It is likely that this is a future of restriction, conflict and unhappiness. Would they be thanking you for 'keeping them safe' and following your rules? It's unlikely isn't it? Think now of the alternative future, where you start and continue in the fight towards an OCD-free life. What will your relationships be like after five or ten years of this? What will you be able to do? How will others feel about you for *not* being obsessional? This is a real choice that you have and a real future that you can have, if you let go of your OCD.

# PARENTS WITH OCD

Spouses, friends and parents are usually the people most involved in supporting people with OCD as they are adults, but in families with children there are some particular issues and questions that often present themselves.

## MY OCD IS MAKING IT VERY DIFFICULT TO DEAL WITH MY CHILD'S DEVELOPMENT AND BEHAVIOUR

As we develop from infancy to adulthood, we all go through a number of different developmental stages. If you are a parent with

OCD, depending on the time that you developed the problem and depending on the type of OCD you have, it is possible that various aspects of your child's behaviour may have come into conflict with the demands and rules of your OCD. One obvious example is, if you have worries about contamination and dirt, then the normal behaviour of a toddler and child – getting very messy, putting their little hands in all sorts of things and in their mouths – may be very anxiety provoking. The OCD may say, 'Well, it's fine to take a risk with yourself, but what about your child?! That's really irresponsible!' This is not true. OCD is a damaging problem that causes people to take unnecessary and *excessive* precautions that become a problem in themselves – your child needs to explore and have contact with the world. The most responsible thing you can do is *not* to do what the OCD wants and to allow the baby to do 'normal things'. It is important to see that the OCD will focus you on one domain, in this example safeguarding the child's physical health. If you think about *all* the things that contribute to being a good parent, there is far more to it than that. Most people would also include emotional availability, ability to have fun, the ability to soothe and comfort the child and many other qualities and abilities. All these things are important (although no one person will be perfect in any domain); focusing on just one part of being a parent is likely to affect the other parts. Fighting back against the OCD will put things back in balance and help you be the best you can be.

If you are not sure what is 'normal' with regard to boundaries for children, have a look when you see parents with their children and ask other parents if you can what sort of approach they take. There will always be a range of behaviour and different opinions on how to go about things. However, most people would not take the extremes of overprotection/restriction of the child or under-protection/laxness but will be somewhere in the middle as a general guide.

Another area that may be difficult for you if you have OCD is helping your child manage their own fears and anxiety, and this is perhaps particularly difficult if your child is showing signs of being obsessional. This is very understandable – of course, it will be harder for you to help your child if their fears chime with yours and many parents with OCD feel very guilty that they may have 'passed on' the OCD (more below). Recent research says that working on your own difficulties will help you help your child as you will truly know what the experience is like and the realities of facing up to your anxiety. Many treatment programmes for children with clinical levels of anxiety will involve the parent as a co-therapist (whether they have anxiety or not). Treatment is likely to be more effective if the parent has at least an understanding of their own difficulties.

## CAN I PASS ON OCD TO MY CHILDREN?

If you have suffered from the debilitating effects of OCD, it is understandable that you will not want your children to experience what you have been through. It is a common worry that OCD can be 'passed on' to children, particularly for parents whose own parent may have had the disorder. Of course, children are influenced by parents, that is the way that it should be, and if you have OCD they may have noticed that you are anxious at times and will try to make sense of that. However, remember that the OCD is only one part of you and what is going on in their lives. We discussed biological and psychological vulnerabilities in more detail in Chapter 2, but the overall message is that it's perfectly possible to have OCD and for your children not to have OCD. In fact, it's also possible to have OCD and be a very good parent. However, that does not mean that you should live with the OCD, far from it. The fact that it is there means that it will be affecting things in some way, like having less time to give to your children (or yourself) or enjoying being with them less due to the depression and anxiety. It may be affecting life in more direct ways such as stopping you going to particular places or doing certain activities.

Apart from getting rid of the OCD (if that's not immediately possible for you), one of the most important things you can do to minimise any possible impact on your children is to not involve them in your obsessions and rituals. This will not only make sure that they do not 'pick up' any obsessional ideas or get frustrated by having to follow obsessional rules, but it will help you challenge your own OCD and see that those rules are really not necessary. As well as being therapeutic for you, it can be a lot of fun for children to be allowed to make a whole lot of mess. You will enjoy being a parent, and your children will enjoy you far more without OCD in your life. The best thing you can do for you and your child is overcome your OCD.

## DISCLOSURE

There is no hard and fast rule about the best time, how, or indeed whether to tell a child at all that you have OCD. This, of course, depends on the particulars of your situation and the age and nature of the child. As one person in their twenties said, 'My mother used to disappear into the bathroom for hours on end. For years I thought she had some sort of drug problem, but one day she sat us down and said that it was OCD and that she went into the bathroom to do her rituals. I was so relieved!'

You know your situation and your child and can make a judgement as to whether disclosure is appropriate and likely to be helpful. Of course, as ever, the best disclosure is that you have had a problem called OCD but you are now working through it and these are the new things that you and your child will now be doing.

## OCD DURING PREGNANCY AND POST-NATALLY

Until recently OCD during pregnancy and after having a baby had received very little research attention. However, recent studies suggest that OCD may be more common at this time than other times in life, with 2–4% of women experiencing clinical levels of symptoms. Some people develop OCD for the first time either during pregnancy or afterwards, while others find that pre-existing symptoms worsen. However, some people can feel better in pregnancy.

Although perinatal OCD, as OCD at other times, can be about anything, most commonly it revolves around significant fear of harm coming to the infant, with worries frequently focused on accidentally harming the child, the child becoming ill or deliberately harming the child. It is important to note that the occasional experience of all of these worries is absolutely *normal* and indeed very common in parents and parents-to-be. However, some people find themselves so distressed that they will take measures to manage their anxiety or prevent their fears coming true. In this way the thoughts and behaviours can interfere significantly with their well-being and their experiences of pregnancy and parenting. This problem can happen to women and men if their partner is pregnant. As with all forms of OCD, it is the extent of and response to the worries, rather than just having them, that becomes the problem.

For example, in pregnancy a woman may be very concerned that something she eats or touches may cause harm to the unborn baby. This may cause her to avoid and restrict foods, places and situations well beyond the recommended guidelines in order to keep as safe as possible, or at least feel that she has done everything in her power to do so. She may spend large amounts of time cleaning and washing and ask those around her to do the same. Women with such concerns may seek excessive reassurance from friends, family and professionals that the baby is developing okay and that her behaviour is 'safe' and will seldom be reassured by the answers given. Post-natally, these concerns may revolve around other illnesses of childhood with mums taking measures such as excessively checking their child when asleep, so that she does not sleep or relax at all herself.

Another common theme of perinatal OCD is thoughts of deliberately harming your own child. After the birth, many parents experience occasional fleeting thoughts that they may deliberately harm their baby, but are able to dismiss these as meaningless. Some women interpret the very fact that they have these thoughts as meaning that they may act on them and become frightened about their potential to harm their child in a moment of madness. They may then, after the birth, avoid contact with the baby or take special measures to stay 'safe' around the child, such as hiding knives and sharp objects in the home.

It may be particularly difficult for mums firstly to recognise their experiences as OCD and then to seek help due to the shame and secrecy associated with the disorder, especially at a time when they and those around them expect them to feel happy. As there is often a lack of awareness of OCD during pregnancy and post-natally, people are rarely asked about these experiences by professionals. If you think that you might have symptoms it may be up to you to suggest that you have OCD and ask for an assessment by someone who knows about this problem.

## HELPING SOMEONE BREAK FREE FROM OCD – INFORMATION FOR FAMILY AND FRIENDS

This section is designed to be read by people who are helping someone trying to break free from OCD. In Chapter 1 we discussed recognising OCD in someone you know and how to approach the problem if you are not sure it is OCD. Here we discuss developing a shared understanding and turning this into strategies for helping someone break free from OCD.

You may be a partner, friend or the son or daughter of someone who has this problem and, if so, it is likely that OCD is affecting you in some way too. In fact it can be *really* hard living with someone who has OCD. At the very least it is upsetting to see someone you care about struggling with the problem and stuck in harmful cycles of behaviour. For most people with OCD, the harm extends beyond themselves: for friends, partners and family, constantly being asked for reassurance, perhaps trying to follow OCD rules and coping with the sufferer avoiding everyday tasks and places can be very draining and can cause lots of conflict. In most cases, the person with OCD knows that their behaviour is excessive and feels very guilty about the impact it is having on others, but even so, they are stuck doing the same things. This is because they really have been stuck in the grip of the OCD bully.

Throughout this book we have encouraged those with OCD to think about how much the problem is affecting all aspects of their life, including relationships. Even though this is sometimes painful to reflect on, we want people to do this so that they can say 'enough is enough' to OCD and stay motivated in the sometimes difficult and uncomfortable job of standing up to this bully.

## GETTING A SHARED UNDERSTANDING OF THE PROBLEM

Of course, only the person who has the problem can do the work of breaking free from OCD, but reading parts of this book or getting the person to explain it to you will give you a deeper understanding of *why* they do what they do. The most important things for friends and family to remember are that:

1. OCD takes a grip when people are stuck in the belief that something bad will happen unless they behave in a certain way (checking, washing or ruminating for example) and it will be their fault if it does.
2. Over time, the behaviours become very damaging, but because they are motivated by the person trying to *prevent harm* and *believing it really could happen*, they feel like they are choosing the lesser of two evils, if they feel that they are choosing at all.
3. Because they are afraid, standing up to OCD takes huge amounts of courage.

A discussion may help them clarify their own understanding of OCD and might also give you the opportunity to ask questions and explain things from your point of view. However, sometimes this sort of discussion is difficult as the topics can be very sensitive – just having a shared general understanding of how OCD works is a good starting point.

## FIGHTING A COMMON ENEMY

People with OCD have spent a long time trying to stop bad things from happening. Throughout this book we present an alternative way of understanding OCD – that it is a problem of worry and anxiety about the meaning of thoughts and about terrible things happening. How one deals with a worry problem is to confront the fears to find out what really happens. In practice, broadly speaking, this means not washing or checking to see what happens, or not grappling with thoughts. It also means not avoiding anything. Although this may be terrifying at first, if someone with this problem can really direct their efforts at beating the problem of worry, the OCD will have nothing to grip on to.

As a supporter, having an understanding not only of what OCD is, but how to deal with it, will be really helpful at those moments when the person is being sucked back into the problem. It may be worth drawing up some strategies together for those times. Some examples are below:

**When I ask you if you washed your hands:**
- Remind me it's OCD and I don't need reassurance
- Delay for 30 minutes and then ask me if I still want reassurance

**When I want to go back to check the locks:**
- Remind me it's just a thought and a good chance to practise standing up to OCD

Remember, it's okay if you both find it hard to stick to these. Just have another go at working out the strategies or getting the sufferer to remember why they are there when they are less anxious.

## WHAT TO ENCOURAGE

It is important to encourage the person to *choose to change* – perhaps remind them what life could be like without this problem, that when things are tough it's just the OCD trying to bully them as it wants to stay around.

Supporting their motivation is useful. Wherever possible, ask them what they are planning to do or what they have done to work on their OCD. Help them recognise when they achieve their goals.

Offer support and encouragement wherever possible – and for yourself too, as supporting someone with this problem takes patience and time.

Rewards help too: perhaps aim for a treat together that OCD may have got in the way of in the past.

## What to avoid

People with OCD are often told to 'just stop' doing their rituals. Blanket bans or strategies like removing the means by which they can do their compulsions (e.g. soap) does not give them a choice and will be experienced as unhelpful.

## Looking after yourself

It's important to remember that it is not your responsibility to cure someone of their OCD, and that you are there to support them in their journey. If you could have done it for them you probably would have! Living with someone with OCD can be a strain and if you are experiencing difficulties, focusing on helping yourself will make you a more effective supporter for them. This could be something simple like making sure you get to do at least some of the activities you want, even if your friend or family member cannot, due to the OCD. It might mean something more like seeking support or even professional help for yourself. Some resources are given at the end of the book, including websites with dedicated sections for supporters.

For people with OCD it can sometimes take a few goes to really get rid of the problem, perhaps because the person is not truly ready to let go at that particular time or there is just too much else going on. Encouraging them to seek help is important and we have more suggestions about this for sufferers in the previous chapter.

# 9
# LIFE AFTER OCD

This chapter gives further guidance on how to continue in your fight against OCD and kick it out of your life for good. We discuss the experience of other difficulties that can be found with OCD and what you might do if you find that this is the case for you.

## RECLAIMING YOUR LIFE

In Chapter 7 we asked you to revisit your goals and remind yourself of what you have to gain by getting rid of the problem. In reality, you have even more to gain as there is a whole future ahead of you that OCD won't have any influence on at all. If you have had OCD for some time, you may not be sure what you would like to have in its place and it is fine not to know. It's also important to begin to find out. If you choose to do something or not do it, it should be because of reasons other than OCD.

It is awful to be stuck in the inward-looking and frightening world of obsessions and compulsions. Getting out of this and engaging with life as it is will always be better than being stuck in OCD's world. Of course, that does not mean that life without OCD is perfect, and breaking free from OCD *may* mean that you need to solve other problems or face up to responsibilities that others have been managing for you when you have been stuck in it. However, not having OCD will give you the time and capacity to deal with these situations. If you have got through a problem like OCD then you have shown strength and a character that you can apply to whatever life throws at you.

Sometimes when people break free from OCD and recover, they feel very sad for all the time they have wasted performing unnecessary rituals, checks and ruminations. It is true that it is very sad to have been doing all those things but this makes it all the more important to continue to kick OCD out permanently and not waste any more time.

# KEEPING OCD AWAY – RELAPSE PREVENTION

If you have taken the courage to fight back against OCD or are even thinking about doing this, then well done. Once you have begun to move on from OCD, it is a common concern that it will come back. Therefore it is important to recognise that you have got better, not by luck or by magic, but through your own efforts, even if you have been working alongside a therapist.

As we have said throughout this book, the way to break free from this problem is to understand as fully as possible how OCD has been working to keep you believing that you are responsible for preventing something bad happening, and then to test this out.

If you have been able to do this, you will have gained information about how the world really works, which is invariably different to what the OCD has been telling you. To do this takes real bravery and it will have felt like a huge risk because OCD is always about what is most important and most dear to people. It is through your hard work in thinking things through, understanding what the OCD is saying, considering an alternative and doing things differently that you have made progress.

It is useful to write up a 'relapse prevention' document. The more you can do to put all that you have learned in one accessible place and think through any situations in the future where the OCD might have a go at you, and what you might think and do in response, the less likely this is to actually happen.

---

**KEY IDEA**

Remember that OCD developed as a way of dealing with difficult thoughts, feelings and circumstances when you did not have any other way of understanding or dealing with it. It is possible that future stressful circumstances may revive an urge to do something obsessional that was perhaps long ago a way of coping. However, what you now know is that this is limited. OCD is a false friend and life is so much better without it. OCD works by keeping you in a mesh of lies and fear that you have already exposed. The reasons you wanted to break free from OCD and the way you did it will provide your blueprint for breaking free if the OCD ever tried to pay you another visit.

---

It is useful to write up a 'relapse prevention' doument or 'blueprint for breaking free'. You can try writing your own blueprint for breaking free using the outline on pages 278 and 279, and the guidance and information from previous chapters.

Jennifer's blueprint is reproduced below:

## JENNIFER'S BLUEPRINT FOR BREAKING FREE

What sort of background factors made me more likely to develop OCD?

*I was always caring and sensitive and worried a great deal about bad things happening and it being my fault. Because of this I was quite protected by my parents.*

How did the problem develop?

*The problem got worse when I went to university and was much more responsible for my actions and I worried about things that weren't in my control. A big trigger was hearing about a fire in a student flat.*

What were the main intrusive thoughts (images/urges/doubts, etc) and what did I think they meant when they were bothering me?

*If I had an image of something bad happening I thought I had to act or they might come true and it would be my fault.*

What do I now know they meant?

*They were just thoughts caused by anxiety, not signs of danger.*

Once the problem took hold, what was it that I was doing, thinking and paying attention to that kept the problem going?

*I started to be more and more aware of anything that might cause a fire and the possibilities were endless. I was trying to be certain that nothing bad would happen but I was seldom able to achieve this, even with more and more time spent checking.*

How did I challenge these and what did I learn? (Describe most useful behavioural experiments and any other way you identified or challenged the processes.)

*I dropped my checks and left the house for increasingly long periods of time.*

*I learnt that I gained confidence in myself and my memory.*

## What were the underlying ideas and beliefs about myself, responsibility or how the world works that kept the problem going?

*I thought that I was a careless person, and that if I wasn't careful something bad would happen. I thought that, knowing this, I needed to put all my effort into preventing this otherwise I would have been responsible for harm.*

## How did I challenge these and what did I learn? (Describe most useful behavioural experiments and any other way you challenged the beliefs.)

*I dropped my checks and left the house for increasingly long periods of time. I learnt that nothing bad happened.*

## What are more helpful versions of those ideas?

*I am a very caring, careful and responsible person and so I really don't need to take extra care.*

*I can tolerate uncertainty and it is not my responsibility to make things 100% safe, even if it were possible!*

*Not being 100% certain is not the same as being 100% unsafe.*

## What can I do now that the OCD was stopping me from doing?

*I am no longer late for everything and I always arrive prepared for lectures.*

*I don't have to think twice about accepting an invitation.*

What can I continue to do to reclaim my life from OCD and beyond?

*Keep doing anti-OCD things, particularly if I feel an urge to check things again.*

What is the best thing about me standing up to OCD?

*I've got my freedom back!*
*I've realised I am a strong person.*

What sort of situations might I find difficult in the future and why? What would I do?

*Exam stress may make me want to take more care and check more. I'll find other ways to deal with the stress – use support from friends, family; balance exercise and relaxation.*

*If I get my own flat – this will be a big responsibility.*

*I will have a copy of this blueprint with me, and act in an anti-OCD way if I feel I need to repeatedly check things again.*

# EPILOGUE

The key to moving on from OCD is to understand as fully as possible how the problem works and how it works for you.

This brings into awareness the fact that OCD is understandable within the context of normal psychological processes. For reasons to do with a person's historical, developmentally acquired experiences and beliefs about the world, as well as a modicum of biological factors, some people are, broadly speaking, much more sensitive to threat. This provides a context for the OCD to take hold, and these are 'vulnerability' factors. Obviously we can't change what has happened to us, and we can't change too much about our biology but we can gain a new understanding of these factors and how they contributed to the problem. If you have had OCD in the past then there may be residues of associations, as would be the case with people with past eating disorders or people who used to smoke heavily. Such people may experience some associations between food or cigarettes and anxiety years after they have beaten their problems, but this does not mean they have relapsed if they do. One of the key facts about OCD is that the occurrence of intrusive thoughts is normal, so getting the occasional one is absolutely within the normal range of experience. If you have been really troubled by intrusive thoughts in the past you can't just forget having had that experience and be like someone who has never had OCD (although you can get very close), but you can apply what you have learnt about the problem to the point of automaticity, and if you keep doing that then the thoughts won't have any hold on you. To be restored to health does not mean not having a past, but we can use our experiences of getting better to stay better.

# RESOURCES

NICE Guidelines for OCD (2005) including full guidelines and version written for patients and carers: http://www.nice.org.uk/CG031

## FURTHER HELP AND SUPPORT WITH OCD

Often people who have OCD, or their friends and families, find it useful to hear about the experiences of others with similar problems. Several websites and self-help organisations exist to promote the understanding and treatment of OCD and provide support and help to sufferers and their families. The main ones in the UK are OCD-UK, OCD Action and Anxiety UK.

**OCD-UK**
PO Box 8955
Nottingham, NG10 9AU
Tel: 0845 120 3778 or email support@ocduk.org
www.ocduk.org

**OCD Action**
Suite 506–507, Davina House
137–149 Goswell Rd
London, EC1V 7ET
Tel: 0845 390 6232
www.ocdaction.org.uk

**Anxiety UK (formerly National Phobics Society)**
Zion Community Resource Centre, 339 Stretford Road,
Hulme, Manchester, M15 4ZY
Tel: 08444 775 774
www.anxietyuk.org.uk

**National Commissioning Group for OCD and BDD – a service for people who have tried lots of therapy previously**
At the time of writing, the National Commissioning Group (NCG) is a network of national services for adults and children who have severe OCD and who have tried several courses of psychological and pharmacological therapy but this has not successfully treated their OCD. NCG services are able to work more intensively and extensively than most other services. Treatment within this service is accessed by referrals from professionals but you can ask to be referred. Further information is found here: http://psychology.iop.kcl.ac.uk/cadat/NCG/ncg_referrers.aspx

## Further help for other issues
**Child anxiety**
*Overcoming Your Child's Fears & Worries* by Cathy Cresswell and Lucy Willetts (Robinson Publishing)

**Autism**
http://www.autism.org.uk/

**Body Dysmorphic Disorder (BDD)**
*Overcoming Body Image Problems including Body Dysmorphic Disorder* by David Veale, Robert Willson and Alex Clarke (Robinson Publishing)

**Depression**
Crisis support: Samaritans
http://www.samaritans.org/
Tel: 08457 90 90 90

**Eating disorders**
Eating Disorders Association: http://www.b-eat.co.uk/Home

**Generalised Anxiety Disorder (GAD)**
*Overcoming Worry* by Mark Freeston and Kevin Meares (Robinson Publishing)

**Health anxiety**
*Overcoming Health Anxiety* by David Veale and Rob Willson (Robinson Publishing)

**Hoarding**
*Compulsive Hoarding and Acquiring: Workbook (Treatments That Work)* by Gail Steketee and Randy O. Frost (OUP US)

**PTSD and experiences of abuse or neglect**
*Overcoming Childhood Trauma* by Helen Kennerley (Robinson Publishing)

**Self-esteem and self-compassion**
*Compassion* edited by Paul Gilbert (Routledge)
*The Compassionate Mind* (Constable) by Professor Paul Gilbert
*Overcoming Low Self-Esteem* by Dr Melanie Fennell (Robinson Publishing)

**Social phobia or Social Anxiety Disorder**
www.social-anxiety.org.uk

## HOW YOU CAN HELP – TAKING PART IN RESEARCH

The information in this book is based on many years of research studies which have aimed to find out more about how OCD works and how best to treat it. This book would not exist without people with OCD giving up their time to assist with this and we would like to take the opportunity to thank all of those people, including the many individuals who have helped us with our own research. The understanding and treatment of OCD can always be improved and so researchers will need people to continue helping us for a long time. If you would like to take part in research, links to ongoing projects can be found on anxiety clinic and university websites and those for anxiety sufferers given above. If you are interested in a project, read the information sheet carefully for the aims and objectives of the study and what is required of you by taking part. Always make sure that the study has been reviewed by a research ethics committee and has been given formal ethical approval (it will have a reference if so). You are always entitled to ask as many questions as you like and to withdraw if you are not completely happy with any aspect of the study.

# APPENDIX

## APPRAISAL OF THOUGHTS

| INTRUSIVE THOUGHT | APPRAISAL: What is the worst thing about having this thought? What does this mean about me as a person to have these thoughts? What is the worst thing that could happen? Does it feel quite (or very) likely? | COMPULSIONS |
| --- | --- | --- |
| | | |

# GOALS

**It is useful to write down your goals:**

- **SHORT-TERM GOALS** (Things I want to change in the next few weeks)
  e.g. go out to the shops, take children to school, have time to read the newspaper

- **MEDIUM-TERM GOALS** (Things I want to change in the next few months)
  e.g. go to a job interview, go on holiday

- **LONG-TERM GOALS** (Things I want to change in the next year or so)
  e.g. move house, have a baby

# BLANK VICIOUS FLOWER DIAGRAM

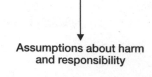

Early experiences

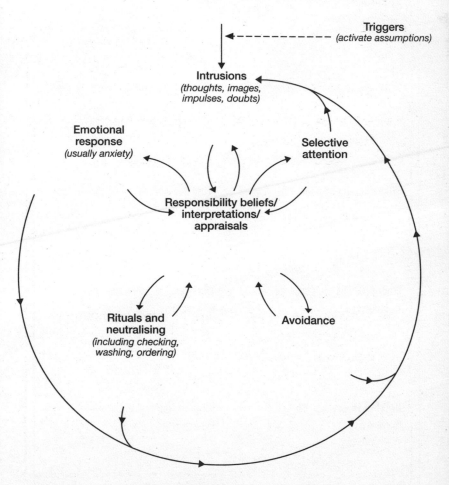

Assumptions about harm
and responsibility

Triggers
*(activate assumptions)*

Intrusions
*(thoughts, images,
impulses, doubts)*

Emotional
response
*(usually anxiety)*

Selective
attention

Responsibility beliefs/
interpretations/
appraisals

Rituals and
neutralising
*(including checking,
washing, ordering)*

Avoidance

# THEORY A AND THEORY B

| THEORY A: OCD SAYS | THEORY B: OCD IS |
|---|---|
| How much do I believe Theory A? (0–100%) | How much do I believe Theory B? (0–100%) |
| Evidence: | Evidence: |
| If this is true, what do I need to do? | If this is true, what do I need to do? |
| What does this say about the future? | What does this say about the future? |
| What does this say about me as a person? | What does this say about me as a person? |
| Belief in Theory A at the end of the exercise | Belief in Theory B at the end of the exercise |

# BEHAVIOURAL EXPERIMENT SHEET

**COMPLETE BEFORE THE EXPERIMENT**

**Planned behavioural experiment**

**Specific predictions and how much I believe them**

**COMPLETE AFTER THE EXPERIMENT**

**Did predictions come true?**

**Conclusions**

**Does this fit best with Theory A or B?**

# BLUEPRINT FOR BREAKING FREE

What sort of background factors made me more likely to develop OCD?


How did the problem develop?


What were the main intrusive thoughts (images/urges/doubts, etc) and what did I think they meant when they were bothering me?


What do I *now* know they meant?


Once the problem took hold, what was it that I was doing, thinking and paying attention to that kept the problem going?


How did I challenge these and what did I learn? (Describe most useful behavioural experiments and any other way you identified or challenged the processes.)


What were the underlying ideas and beliefs about myself, responsibility or how the world works that kept the problem going?

How did I challenge these and what did I learn? (Describe most useful behavioural experiments and any other way you challenged the beliefs.)

What are more helpful versions of those ideas?

What can I do now that the OCD was stopping me from doing?

What can I continue to do to reclaim my life from OCD and beyond?

What is the best thing about me standing up to OCD?

What sort of situations might I find difficult in the future and why? What would I do?

How will I tackle this?
- Possible future difficult situations

- What OCD may tell me

- What I can reply and do

# INDEX